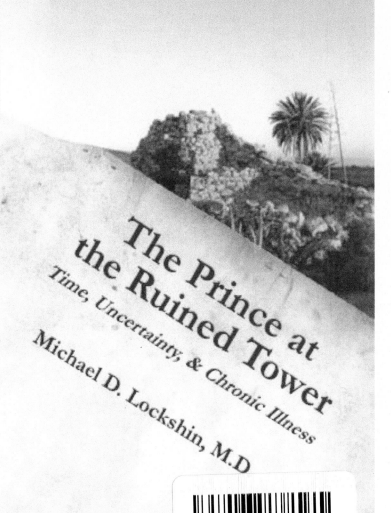

The Prince at the Ruined Tower

Time, Uncertainty, & Chronic Illness

Michael D. Lockshin, M.D

D1214103

The Prince at the Ruined Tower

Time, Uncertainty & Chronic Illness

Michael D. Lockshin, M.D.

First Edition
Custom Databanks, Inc.
New York, NY 10022
www.CustomDatabanks.com

Author photo: The Hospital for Special Surgery
Cover photo: Miriam Lockshin

Paperback Edition
ISBN: 13: 978-1-889782-04-1
ISBN-10:1-889782-04-1

Mobi eBook Edition
ISBN-13: 978-1-889782-05-8
ISBN-10:1-889782-05-X

ePub eBook Edition
ISBN-13: 978-1-889782-06-5
ISBN-10:1-889782-06-8

Dedication

To Jane, the love of my life for the whole of my sentient life, without whom there would not be these ideas nor this book.

Contents

Prologue

For a long time my word meant everything. Standing at a bedside, I pronounced a diagnosis. Debate would then end.

Medical students gathered round, listening to me pontificate. I spoke sagely (I thought) about my patient's perhaps rare, certainly interesting, and often difficult diagnosis. The patient, too, might listen, anxiously, as I dictated, to my students and to her, my ideas about her care.

Looking back, these long ago bedside scenes are like mini-dramas of stage or television, the *leitmotif* of which is my certainty.

There was fog; it will now clear, I had said. There was mystery; it will now be solved. This is the diagnosis. And the prognosis? Well, the timeframe is imprecise, a month, a year, but certainly, I declared, this illness will be gone, or that one will progress. The details might change, but the message was always: The answer will be clear.

I did not accept—could not conceive—the immense space that uncertainty inhabits within the borders of my medical world. Instead I believed that, if one has enough imagination, studies intensely enough, and asks the right questions, there is always a correct diagnosis, prognosis, and cure. The first goal is to name the diagnosis.

If I had allowed uncertainty a place in my discourse I would have thought I had done wrong. In the late twentieth century and at the beginning of the twenty-first, I thought, sometimes said out loud, our knowledge is exceedingly great. How can we *not* know?

I am less arrogant today. I now accept that uncertainty occupies a substantial part of the world in which my patients, my students, and I live. We do not need to hide it from view. It is not cause for fright. Uncertainty is just another tool that we can learn to use.

How did I learn to accept uncertainty?

I used to think that if I did not understand a diagnosis the problem lay in me—an unconfident student's normal fear. Later, when I was a resident physician answering interns' questions, a young professor replying to students, or a doctor talking to patients, I began to think that some of my answers were superficial. I said to myself, as I rambled on, when this conversation ends I will ask a more experienced colleague, or I will re-read the relevant scientific papers, because I am uncertain that the glib answer I just gave is precisely true.

One later day, oblivious to personal growth, standing before a group of students or behind a lectern in a hall, I was surprised to see the audience's eyes directed to me, expectant, asking for clear answers. Asking for certainty from me!

The moment was surreal. I suddenly saw that they deemed my words "authoritative", a not completely bizarre circumstance, because by this time I had talked to, and sometimes collaborated with, luminaries who were the sources of the information that I now shared. I had attended professional meetings and had sat on committees. Perhaps I did have authority for the (small, transient) topic at hand.

I also intuited what I did not know. Formulating a reply to a question, I felt compelled to follow my answer with this disclosure: "And this is what we do not know. The greater story is the uncertainty that remains."

Uncertainty? Everything we hear and read in news stories, in medical textbooks, and in lectures from professors like me, says that medicine has great knowledge. True, if you ignore the obvious: Although yesterday we knew much less, tomorrow we will know much more. We continue to add to our knowledge. Today is a very small point on a very long line of Time. There is always more to learn.

How did I come to embrace uncertainty? Not from my professors. My patients taught this lesson to me.

Patients taught me? Teaching her doctor is not a patient's goal. A patient wants clarity, wants us to solve problems, predict futures, and make her well. A patient does not want to hear that her doctor does not know.

Unpredictability of human illness is the source of the lesson. Doctors set and live by clear-cut rules, but illnesses ignore these rules. This patient's symptoms are too subtle to assign a diagnosis name. That patient's symptoms change with passing time; those of another combine elements of multiple ills and reconstitute themselves in unrecognizable ways.

According to doctors' rules, diagnosis implies treatment and treatment implies cure. It is different in the world of chronic illness: Doctors ameliorate, not cure. We monitor changes that take decades to be seen. Illnesses advance and withdraw in unpredictable ways. Patients, students, and trainees ask me why.

Trying to explain the inexplicable, I begin to think about uncertainty.

How then to share this concept? Do we talk about our uncertainties with the patient, or do we keep them to ourselves? No public forum addresses this concern.

In this book, I pose the question to you. We will have a conversation and decide together what to do.

* * * * *

I make my points by using patients' stories. The stories include passion and anguish and anger, sourced in a patient's pain, and disability, or frustration. My own anger may show through; it finds its origins in the organizational flaws that at times constrain imagination and contradict logical thought. I tell my patients' stories from my point of view. If I have misunderstood their messages, I apologize. I hope someone else will speak on their behalf.

In Part I of this book I talk about how patients, doctors, and administrative systems respond to uncertainty of diagnosis. What happens when patients fit no conventional nosology; when their symptoms and laboratory tests contradict one another; when diagnoses change over time; or when precision molecular diagnoses adds no meaning to a patient's care?

Part II examines uncertainty's boundaries. When doctors disagree about basic facts, is that error or is it uncertainty? What if they agree about the facts but disagree about what they should do? What happens when acknowledging uncertainty does not relieve a patient's pain? How does one proceed when patients demand certainty that the doctor cannot provide?

Part III is about Time: How diagnoses and doctors' concepts change over decades. Part III also describes sums of the circumstantial socioeconomic and biological factors that bring one individual patient to one specific practice site at one specific time, and how a different set of circumstances might lead to a different result.

Part IV considers how organizational constraints of modern American medicine presume a degree of certainty impossible to achieve and thereby threatens the honesty required for mutual trust.

In Part V I discuss how we prioritize facts to make a diagnosis, some of us relying on basic science, others on humanistic features, still others on both. This foray into philosophy contrasts the insights and the deceptions imparted by animal models of human illness; the *how* of an illness compared to its *why*; and how qualitative *versus* qualitative thinking differently describe illness. The melding of these conflicting ideas puts the concept of uncertainty into words, though uncertainty does not need articulation—it can be conveyed non-verbally. One can hear music in the words (a thought that came to me as I read a commentary on an obscure French poem, a thought that gives the title to this book).

Part VI concludes with a roadmap for doctor, patient, student, and public to talk about uncertainty, to define it, to measure it, and to use it as a tool. If I can successfully convey the nature of this journey, we will share a common language.

We can begin our conversation. Let the journey begin.

Part I. Uncertain Diagnosis

1. The Journey Begins

When I was a very young doctor I exuded certainty. Now older, more humble, and less certain, I began to share with those around me my thoughts about uncertainty. My first audiences were my patients and students. I had taught four lessons.

Lesson 1. The key to everything is to make a correct diagnosis. Corollary: Making a correct diagnosis is easy when laboratory tests are abnormal.

Lesson 2. If laboratory tests do not show what the doctor expects, do more tests.

Lesson 3. The key to making a correct diagnosis is to structure every question so that its answer is binary, either *yes* or *no*. If the first answer is *no*, ask another question and, if necessary another, and another. Continue with binary questions until you reach a final *yes*. Stop at that *yes*.

Lesson 4. When you know the diagnosis you know the prognosis. Your patient will get better, or worse, or will stay the same. You also know that the diagnosis will not change.

In fact, belief in the stability of diagnosis is so secure that a doctor, asking a new patient, "What diagnoses have been made before?"—trusts the answer, and does not ask, "What is a diagnosis?" or, "If the patient had X diagnosis several years before, can it have changed to Y?"

When Milagros, a 20-something, newly married, quiet, and modest Nuyorican,[1] a teacher of English as a second language, fell ill, she came to our hospital's emergency room. The ER doctors asked us to assist in her care.

In just a short time—she had been well only a few weeks before—her kidneys failed, her body filled with fluid, her urine stopped flowing, and, the ER doctors had just learned, her blood chemistry tests indicated an immediate threat to her life. If we did not start kidney dialysis at once, Milagros would almost certainly soon die.

This was medical certainty. We knew exactly what to do. We started dialysis immediately, placed big needles into her arms, ran her blood through a big and noisy machine, and spent the next many hours washing

---

[1] A sardonic New York slang term for a New Yorker of Puerto Rican heritage.

the poisons from her blood. Once this was done her life was no longer at risk—for the short term.

Our next challenge was to learn why her kidneys had failed. We would now have to think of the long term to prevent it happening again.

We made a diagnosis, and I then opined that her kidneys would not recover. I predicted that, without a kidney transplant, she would depend on dialysis for the rest of her life. Nonetheless, we, or rather she, had little to lose if we made heroic efforts (the heroism was hers, not ours) to force her kidneys to work again. We prescribed powerful medicines to stop the inflammation that had caused her kidneys to fail, to reverse the process and to let her kidneys heal (if possible). We had little optimism. Reversal of advanced kidney failure of this type is rare.

A few days later, at her bedside with my students, I was certain, and I pontificated. It was all very clear. Her symptoms, blood tests, and a kidney biopsy had shown lupus in its acute and most dangerous form.[2] I know this disease. One might say I know a lot about this disease. So I was confident, as I stood at Milagros' bedside that day, that I knew where this was going to go.

---

[2] Lupus is a common, chronic rheumatic illness that primarily affects young women, and one on which I have spent my career.

My memory is imprecise about the details. On that day long ago I almost certainly announced a bad prognosis. The kidneys would not recover, I would have said. Milagros would depend on dialysis but probably would survive, I would have said. The positive message would have been that, with luck, we could consider a kidney transplant in several years. I would not have been ambiguous. My answers to her questions and to those asked by the students would have been very clear.

I was wrong, of course.

In Spanish the word milagros *means "miracles," a most apposite name.*

After a few months Milagros' kidneys did regain their function. After one year, we removed the dialysis tubes from her arm. A few years later she carried and delivered a healthy daughter, a few years later, another. This all happened long ago, when Milagros and I were both young. Her daughters are now grown. Milagros became principal of her school, then supervisor for several schools. Today she is mostly well. Today I am a more humble man.

My prediction was wrong, but there were more lessons for me to learn. I did not understand then, as now I do, that certainty also implies confidence that what is true today will always be true, that today's wisdom accurately predicts the long term. The day Milagros and I met I was certain of her diagnosis and thus its prognosis. I was certain that I knew how it would evolve. I was wrong on both counts.

Twenty years later Milagros fell ill again, as her disease returned.

I say her disease returned, but other doctors might say that this time she had a different diagnosis because the illness came back in a different form. Her kidneys were now fine; she had severe arthritis. Her blood tests now showed rheumatoid arthritis, a closely related but very different disease.

One diagnosis, or two? Lupus twenty years before, rheumatoid arthritis today? Although the two diseases are similar, I do not like coincidences. More likely, in Milagros, lupus had merely changed its form.

I say one disease had changed its form because it stayed as rheumatoid arthritis for only a few years, then her symptoms vanished and her blood tests became normal again. Then, after another few years, her blood tests showed lupus once more, though she remained well. Several more years passed before symptoms of lupus recurred, then vanished, and her blood tests returned to normal. Today the tests show both diseases, her symptoms are of rheumatoid arthritis alone, and she receives treatment for both.

It was not supposed to be this way. The textbooks tell us that in lupus the kidneys do not recover the way Milagros' did. The textbooks say that lupus and rheumatoid arthritis are separate diseases. Our science says that, though they are closely related, they are distinct from one another. But textbooks do not describe patients like Milagros, in whom lupus and arthritis change from one to the other and then change back again. Milagros' illness paid no attention to our rules.

So what do I conclude now? *Estos son los milagros*, I say. These are miracles. Biology will do what it will do. Textbooks describe only what the doctor who wrote the relevant chapter has himself seen, not what other doctors will later see. If we believe that what we know now is nearly all we will ever know, we will be unable to imagine the surprises tomorrow will bring.

To be clear, Milagros' current good health is due neither to the treatment I first prescribed nor to that which I later gave. I attribute her initial recovery, and the later changes in course that occurred, to *los milagros*. Her illness, setting its own rules, taught me how little I know.

I was certain on that day I first met Milagros. I am less certain today. I now understand, but I did not then, that our twenty-first century concepts of diagnosis are temporary. We cite our past experience; we know generalities. But we cannot know how a diagnosis will progress in any one person. A diagnosis is a descriptive label, nothing more. What we call prognoses, for an individual or for the crowd, are guesses valid only for the short term. Yes, in most cases I can reasonably predict the next year or two or five, but to see decades ahead is beyond my power.

On some future day, a doctor will talk to medical students about the biology of Milagros' diagnosis. Aided by the knowledge that accrues with time, perhaps that future doctor will understand why, in her, lupus disappeared, returned as arthritis, then came and went at will, the miracles, *los milagros*. I can picture that doctor and that bedside scene, but I wonder: Will that future doctor be humble enough to know that in her or his future there will be new biologies that he or she does not at the moment understand? Will that future doctor see the uncertainty that lies ahead?

2. The Tree and the Fairy Ring

Miracles. Prognoses that are wrong. Diagnoses that change over time. How can we be certain about what we know?

Medical textbooks say it is easy to make a clear diagnosis. With great clarity, textbooks tell us the major characteristics of every disease. Each chapter, every medical school lecture, indeed most bedside teaching conversations, say that the first need is to define the patient's diagnosis.

Medical textbook chapters and doctors' lectures have a standard structure: Name the diagnosis. Describe its cause. Explain how it occurs in a population. Illustrate its symptoms, physical examination findings, and laboratory tests. Note its treatment and prognosis. And, sometimes, when the focus of the chapter or lecture is "academic," discuss its deep biology.

What would the title of the chapter be—in what section of the book would it fall?—about an illness as bizarre as that of Milagros, that has no name and fits no rules? And what would the chapter's content be if the author could foresee how one diagnosis would change to another then back again over three decades?

Textbooks tell doctors and patients what they need to know about diagnoses that have names. If the texts are not enough, one can find the answer on the Internet. I tell my students, "Just Google it. An answer will be found." But the answers one finds on Google mislead.[i]

To reach a diagnosis, we are taught and I teach, ask binary questions that can be answered with a *yes* or a *no*. The patient's symptoms are like a tree, doctors are wont to say. The trunk contains general possibilities, like fever or weight loss or pain. Each branch is like a *yes* and *no* answer. Call the trunk fever; the large branches might be infection (if *yes*, follow that branch), tumor, sunstroke, or autoimmune disease (follow other branches). You suspect infection. Do a test. If the test is positive, take the next branch; if negative, take another. Follow the *yes* answers to the smallest branches. If you see only *no* answers, do more tests. At the end of smallest branch, the leaf is your final answer. Now you know which medicine to prescribe.

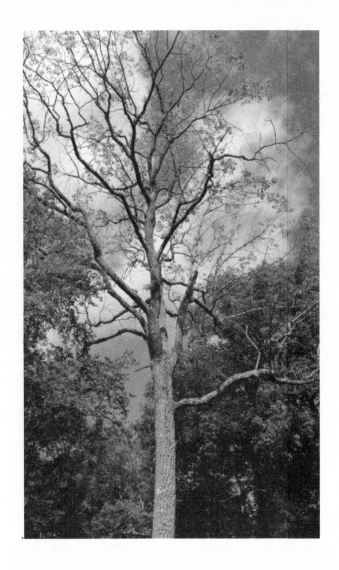

The Branches of a Tree (MDL photo)

In the model of the tree, branches lead in only one direction, getting smaller but more specific each time. At each divide, one branch becomes *yes*, the other *no*. There is no *maybe* branch between. The branches do not rejoin others nor do they turn back toward the trunk. The diagnostic tree has one logic: Trunk divides to large branches, large branches divide to intermediate, intermediate to small, and the last divide is to leaves. One direction. A clear end.

Perhaps at the end of time the tree model may at last be true, with a single, unequivocal leaf always at the end. It is not true today, at least not for chronic disease.

A better model might be this: Instead of the tree, tall and assertive in forest or plain, think of diagnosis as a mushroom fairy ring.

Do you not know what this is? Walk in a temperate forest in late summer. Look at what is visible low on the ground. On occasion you will see mushrooms lined up in a neat row.

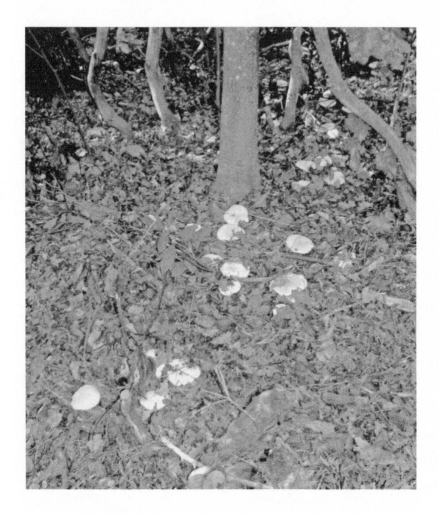

A Mushroom Fairy Ring (MDL photo)

If the forest is not too dense, and if your eyes follow that row, you will see that it forms a gentle curve, an arc of a large circle, and you will understand: There must be an underlying plan.

And what might that plan be?

It is that the mushrooms of this ring are the fruits of an enormous plant, called a mycelial network, that lies beneath the soil. When the plant is ready to seed, it pushes its flower (the mushrooms) through the earth, but only at its edge, showing only the network's outline, like a thin frame about a painting or a low fence about a yard, a *soupçon* of a great mass below.

A fairy ring is the external sign of a network of roots that spread unseen below. Those roots join and rejoin and turn backward and go forward and up and down in a mesh that defies delineation, its direction impossible to know. The fairy ring is a metaphor for some patients' symptoms: Eternally visible parts that may seem insignificant but instead hint at great complexity, of a much larger process that connects them all.

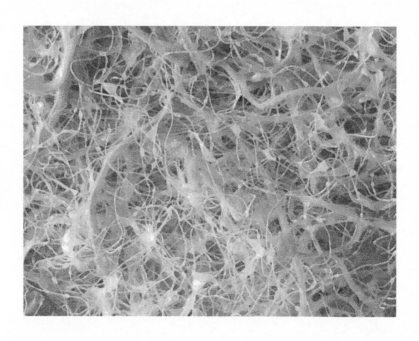

A Mycelial Network (the mushrooms' roots)

3. Acute, Chronic

A tree dominant on the horizon. A mushroom ring hinting about a great unseen network below. These are also metaphors for the thinking patterns doctors use. They are metaphors for acute and chronic disease.

Acute illness is immediate, dominant, and unsubtle like the tree. Pain? Fever? Seizure? Fracture? Answers about acute illness, like those of the tree, are straightforward and binary. A large branch has rot (an abscess): Cut the rot out. Wind cracked a branch (a fracture, of tree or bone): Treat it with a splint or a nail. The problems of acute illness are finite. They occupy a small piece of space and not much time. They require no deep knowledge or search for hidden things. Identify the problem, take precise, aggressive action—excise the rot, bolt the branch; splint the fracture, drain the abscess, give an antibiotic—and effect a definitive repair. That is acute illness.

Chronic illness is like the mushroom ring. It is the set of symptoms, some coordinate and some seemingly independent of one another, but all markers of a problem, the part easy to mistake for the whole. Doctors will differ in how they respond to these hints. Some will see only the ring; uncurious, they will focus on, and treat, only the distinct symptoms—lower the temperature, relieve the pain—thinking this will suffice, and not see the hidden, possibly lethal, part that remains intact and sound. More thoughtful doctors will intuit the unseen network, try to trace its many directions, hunting for its core. Pluck the mushroom, the mycelial network remains. Contain it, dig it out, effect some form of control—that is the better way.

This is what doctors do not teach, what administrators ignore, and what patients rarely understand: Acute illness differs from chronic. One is a tree, the other a mushroom fairy ring. Confronting one, confronting the other, doctors and their patients will exercise different thinking processes, and they will have different goals.

We rarely speak of the difference between acute and chronic illness today, but we once did. People from generations past use to say, "I have a condition, not a disease," by which they meant a chronic or an acute illness. A condition, the chronic, implied permanence; a disease implored transience, with expectation of cure or of death.

My grandparents' generation understood this: In their time (and in ours) patients went to doctors, often unexpectedly, often urgently, for *treatment* of acute episodes of ill health. As a rule, acute illnesses have few antecedents. They come by surprise. Once treated, they will be gone. Acute illnesses have high personal drama, involve strangers—ambulance attendants, emergency room personnel. Acutely ill patients expect immediate interventions and cures, the rot cut off, the injury repaired.

People with chronic illnesses go, usually by prior plan, usually electively, for *management* of conditions. They go to doctors' offices by appointment and with little drama. They come alone, or sometimes with a spouse or relative or friend. Often the first symptom is ambiguous, just a hint of something wrong, barely enough to notice, but it gradually grows, perhaps spreads to other areas, perhaps becomes more intense. Sometimes it comes for a while, disappears, and then returns. Often the patient has suspected for a long time that something is wrong. The diagnosis may be obvious at the time of the visit or it may require time to evolve. Its symptoms might be below the threshold that allows a doctor to assign a name.

Once aware of the meaning of chronicity, patients lower their expectations. Immediately for some, slowly for others, they begin to understand that, for them, the goal may be amelioration, not cure. The patient may not understand this on a first or second visit. She may not yet know that relief of pain or prevention of disability, not cure, will be the doctor's goal. My grandparents knew this difference.

The word *diagnosis*, and the way we use it, makes no distinction between acute and chronic. Administrators and doctors wrongly assume that treatment and management of either use the same rules. Acute illness is what television dramas and the popular press portray as what doctors do. Acute illness is what is known to the ER.

This is not the world of which I speak. My world is that of chronic illness, which lacks the certainty of unequivocal diagnosis and cure. In my world time passes and facts change. Once believed certain, assumptions need to be revised. In the world of chronic illness, pathways merge and intertwine in hidden networks, like the underground network that reveals itself only to those imaginative enough intuit the fairy ring. Acute illness' model is simplicity. That of chronic illness is complexity.

4. Uncertainty: Anna and Dale

We doctors expend great effort to give descriptive or obfuscating (should that be descriptive *and* obfuscating?) names—we call them diagnoses—to the many bodily woes that beset mankind, but diagnoses do not read our textbooks. Indeed, we base our reputations, our claims to knowledge of deep things, our demand for high respect and for high recompense, on our ability to assign difficult-to-pronounce names, names so complex that they imply wisdom, to symptoms that fail to follow the rules that our certainty in giving them these names requires.

We give names to rashes and pains and fevers. We note that one body system or another works normally, or abnormally, or not at all. We do blood tests and take pictures and thread tubes into various places so that we can precisely label (not necessarily fix) what has gone wrong. We find microbes and viruses and even genes that threaten our health. If we do these things well, we make it possible to find a corrective treatment, administer it, and make you well.

This is the reigning paradigm. One set of symptoms, one pattern of laboratory tests, one set of X-ray images: One diagnosis name. A different set, a different diagnosis.

We doctors seldom discuss what to do when the pattern does not match the chosen name. We usually assume that the information base is true and that someone has made a mistake. Our observations were careful, thoughtful, and insightful, we had thought, but perhaps the observations were wrong. Did Milagros have several sequential diagnoses, or, more likely, was the true one initially missed and became obvious later on—that's what the paradigm would say—or was the first diagnosis correct but it changed its form over time, an assertion that contradicts the paradigm? What does one say when symptoms of several diagnoses occur in the same person at the same time? What does one say if you suspect that the information base is false, and that no textbook chapter accurately describes what any doctor's eyes can see?

Early one summer I met two ill young women, Anna just before Memorial Day, Dale six weeks after that. Both seemed to have many diseases together. The doctors they had seen before, each in turn, had tried to narrow the possible diagnoses to a single name. After all, they are both so young, how could they have more than one disease?

For both patients, the different doctors disagreed on what that choice should be. Diagnosis A, said one; diagnosis B, said another, then diagnosis C or diagnosis D. The confusion, the inability to select just one diagnosis, made their parents and the young ladies anxious. Their doctors, one after the other, hesitated to start treatment until they knew the correct name. When they suggested treatments, they, of course, disagreed.

Anna's parents first, then Dale's, presented their daughters to me. My job as a consultant, they said, is to choose among the offered diagnoses so that the appropriate treatment can begin. For both women the choices were the same: Lupus, scleroderma, Sjögren's disease, lymphoma, cryoglobulinemia, or dermatomyositis. I know you find that complicated, but the diseases have many similarities of both symptoms and laboratory tests. It is not unusual for doctors to become confused.

I had examined Anna and I examined Dale. I did more tests. At the conclusion of both consultations I found that I had no idea which name to use.

That was not ignorance. I concluded that the name did not matter. A name is only a simple description, invented by humans, that describes an appearance that may not reflect the core. It is a mnemonic, a mushroom ring that hints at complexity below. A name is a label for a process that we may, but often do not, understand. The process is what determines a person's fate, not the name.

We give diseases names that seem right today. Long ago, although the same diseases had different names, the processes were still the same. Doctors once spoke of ague; today we speak of fever and chills. Our forebears diagnosed milk leg, today thrombophlebitis, a blood clot in a leg that occurs after childbirth. They gave names to symptoms: Dropsy (accumulation of fluid), or consumption (decay). Today we give names to the processes (as we understand them) that cause those symptoms: Heart failure, tuberculosis. Dropsy or heart failure, the patient's abdomen and legs still swell. Consumption or tuberculosis, he still coughs. In the future, with better tools, we will discover new processes that will stratify groups of symptoms in different ways. We will invent new diagnosis names. In 1916 and 2016 and 2116 the names were, are, and will be different, but the boil will still drain, the cancer still invade, the blood vessel still become blocked, in the same way as it did in 2016 BCE and today, and as it will in centuries to come.

So for Anna and for Dale the answer to "What is my diagnosis?" is: "On this day, in this place, we use this name."

Even when the name fairly describes the biological process that we call a disease, what do we learn when we use that name?

Within the context of the name patients differ. Some with a straight-forward, unambiguous diagnosis are barely touched by the illness and need no treatment at all. Others with the same diagnosis are lethally ill. For some patients the illness appears and vanishes in a week or two; for others it lingers on.

I do not believe in coincidence. I do not believe that Anna and Dale have several simultaneous but similar diagnoses. Parsimoniously I conclude that each has just one illness, or one process, that makes them ill. The confusion comes from the fact that our contemporary understanding of the process does not explain how the symptoms are linked. If I were forced to choose and therefore act just one diagnosis name, as that name is understood today, I would have to ignore an accumulating pile of inconvenient facts. I would have no flexibility to rethink the problem at some future time.

Single diagnosis names work for average patients, "classical" patients who have all of a disease's features, but it does not work for Anna and Dale. So how important is the name?

In theory, we use diagnosis names to predict a patient's outcome and to direct treatment. Because patients like Anna and Dale are not rare, and because severity of symptoms within a single diagnosis name may range from nil to lethal, today's names fail at their assigned tasks. Thoughtful doctors note, but are not constrained by, a diagnosis name. They make new choices when circumstances change. Unthoughtful doctors adhere to the single diagnosis name and treat formulaically, by rote.

Whether today I do or do not assign a label to the process that afflicts Anna or Dale will make no difference for their future lives. I will still treat them for what I see. To the contrary, if I become beholden to the name I have chosen, and if I treat solely on the basis of that belief, and do not acknowledge the anomalies within, I may do more harm than good.

On those days in that early summer I did not give either woman a diagnosis name, nor did I continue to do tests to fulfill that intellectual and administrative need. Instead, I told them and their parents that it was important to find those parts of the puzzle that I do know how to treat. The information they brought from their other doctors and that I now had was sufficient. Now, I said, is time to be open-minded and flexible, to accept uncertainty about a diagnosis name, and to act on the treatable process abnormalities that are certain today.

5. The "Certainty" of Google

Accept uncertainty? When one can quickly find answers for every question on the Internet? In an era when it is so easy to query the world?

When my wife and I debate the day's news at dinner, questions arise. Where exactly is Andorra? In what book did X say Y? Few of our dinner table debates move forward without one of us saying that the question just asked is a Google Opportunity. Then we reach for the smart-phones or tablets, competing to find the answer.

Here is a sample of this week's queries: The biographical details of an author, a review of whose new book I have just read. Maps of Paris and Boston. Driving instructions to a country house to which we have been invited to lunch. The origin of a strange name of a television actress. Translations of various terms from several languages. Verification of a literary citation. Geography of the Caucasus. Names of states ending in *–istan*. Almost any assertion that anyone makes these days is subject to a challenge that can be immediately answered on Google or its rivals.

Except in the world of chronic illness.

Of course there are Internet sites about illnesses. Of course best treatments (according to the diagnosis) are listed. But how do you search answers for Anna or Dale, whose diagnoses have no correct name? You cannot logically search for multiple diagnoses that occur simultaneously. You cannot ask how, or for how long, diagnoses change over time. How do you query symptoms that do not match physical findings or for laboratory tests that match no symptoms? Can Google explain the changing pattern of Milagros' disease? Can Google trace the intertwining, intersecting, coalescing, regressing, and progressing line of the complex network hiding below the mushroom ring?

The world of acute illness is different. Doctors who treat acute illness less willingly accept uncertainty. They make rapid, clear decisions. Is it a heart attack? Do a blood test or an electrocardiogram. The answer is *yes* or *no*. The heart's rhythm is normal or it is not, and when it is not, here is a drug that fixes it. Is it pneumonia? The X-ray says *yes* or *no*. If *yes*, here is an antibiotic. Is it trauma? Here is a cast for your fracture. In acute illness patient and doctor are together only for a short time. Their interactions have a beginning, a middle, and an end. Nothing is vague. At the end of the encounter, no questions remain.

In the world of chronic illness, the time scales are long, and interactions take place over months and years. Pain and swelling come and go, start in one part of the body, go to another, then move to still another. Over extended time symptoms change. Ill for one week, well for a month, then ill again. Flare-ups and then remissions. To discover the meaning of the symptoms requires watching, adjusting, and rethinking as the symptoms change. Observing, and not intervening, is often a very good choice. Sometimes the changing pattern gives a clue. Sometimes the manner in which a patient does or does not respond to a specific treatment is a clue. To wait, to watch, to try something specific and observe the response—this is the world of uncertainty.

Ambiguity about diagnosis causes anxiety for both patients and doctors. Driven by unease, some doctors, and some patients, enter an unending and often fruitless quest for clarity. They continue in their search for the elusive *yes*. Sometimes their hunt succeeds. If it does, the next question is: Was the search worthwhile? Now that we have a name, was anything gained?

I imagine that the sun was bright and the temperature high in that faraway place, on that late November day, when Amirah boarded the airplane that brought her to New York.

The city she left is in one of those small, distant, desert countries, the name of which evokes images of sand and oil, as well as queries about where to find it on a map. It is a place at a great geographic and cultural remove. From desert sun to snowbound town, after fourteen hours in the air, Amirah's flight landed in New York, as she sought to find a name for her diagnosis.

At first glance the details were straightforward. Her vision had become blurred, her right arm and leg had become weak, and she staggered when she walked. She and the doctors in her distant land thought it relevant that she had lost eight pregnancies in a row. She wanted a diagnosis, health regained, and the chance to have a healthy child.

Her local doctors had found two abnormal antibodies in her blood. One suggested a disease similar to multiple sclerosis; another suggested Sjögren's syndrome, an autoimmune disease that can affect the brain. Her doctors were confused, she said. They advised her—or perhaps she decided on her own—to seek an opinion in America. It was hard to be certain of all the details. We talked through a translator, and not all points were clear. Because of her culture's norms, she did not look directly to my eyes. Although she spoke calmly, Amirah's eyes showed fear.

As with Anna and Dale, I thought that Amirah's multiple problems—gait, vision, and pregnancy losses—derived from one, not several, disease processes. I thought the primary problem was autoimmune, hence in my field, but I would not give her illness a name. How does one translate ambiguity? I could not tell whether she understood.

Amirah came to New York to see several doctors, not just me. A neurologist agreed with me: It was a type of brain inflammation. Discounting the abnormal antibodies, a second neurologist offered a different idea, too much pressure on the brain. He admitted her to the hospital for a procedure that would remove excess spinal fluid to bring down the pressure on the brain.

These consultations and the hospitalization took place during the Christmas season. After arranging for Amirah's hospital admission, the second neurologist went on holiday, and I, too, was away. Because of the holidays, the neurology team that covered the second neurologist rotated attending (in-charge) physicians each day, so a different neurologist saw her on each of Amirah's six inpatient days. Neither I nor the physician covering me had been told that she was in the hospital, so I had no advice to give. The story below comes from the hospital chart notes that I read after I returned.

Hospital rules require a daily progress note to be written by the attending physician. That daily note must include a diagnosis and a plan. Thus the six different neurologists, on six successive days, recorded the following diagnoses in Amirah's chart: Sjögren's syndrome, increased pressure on the brain, multiple sclerosis, increased pressure, depression, multiple sclerosis. Not one of the notes suggested the possibility that the diagnosis was ambiguous. By the evidence of their notes, each neurologist was certain.[3]

She had visible symptoms, but they were not rapidly progressing, in fact were rather stable from one day to the next, so each neurologist thought it wise to postpone treatment until the neurologist who had admitted her returned from his holiday. I came back before he did. Amirah, now an outpatient again, came to my office and asked me to explain.

The new information from the hospital chart did not change my original opinion. Through the translator I tried to explain to Amirah: "These tests are positive, and these others are not. I believe that the process is autoimmune. Although many diagnoses are possible, I cannot give you a single diagnosis name. I do have a good idea what will happen to you, and I do know what to do."

---

[3] The issue concerning a doctor's need to be unambiguous is partly due to a doctor's personal beliefs but is also due to an administrative requirement for writing precise code numbers for diagnoses to justify test requisitions and treatment plans. If ambiguity is implied, permission to do tests and payments for all aspects of care will be denied by insurers. I discuss this issue later in this book. In this specific case, I am talking about the chart notes themselves, which, as written, supported the diagnostic codes that had been assigned.

I think that was the only true answer, ambiguous but not a lie. Yes, she was frightened. Truth be told, some of the covering doctors had seemed more frightened than she.

I began the treatment I favored and she improved. Two months later it was time for her to return to her home. She had come to New York to learn these things: That she was not lethally ill, that another pregnancy would be safe, that the illness would likely not progress, and that we did have a treatment plan. I had given her those answers. She had also asked for, but it seemed to me that, she no longer required, a diagnosis name. She accepted that I would not answer that final question. Through the translator, she told me that she could live with the uncertainty, so long as she knew I had a plan.

On the morning of the day she was to leave, she came to my office to collect a summary for the doctors in her country and to say goodbye. As she walked out the door I told her once again through the translator, "This is what I believe will happen."

She stopped abruptly and then turned back. Uncharacteristically, she looked straight into my eyes.

"Insha'Allah," she said.

I do not speak Arabic, but that was easy to understand.

"Yes, of course," returning her gaze, I replied, "Insha'Allah."

6.   Diagnoses That Are Too Clear

The symptoms of rheumatic diseases often begin quietly, evolve slowly, and are vague. "I ache all over." Or, "I am tired all the time." Or, "I feel like I have a fever, or the flu." Or (patients often say), "I'm so young but I feel so old." They do not recognize, or dismiss the possibility, that they may be seriously ill.

Symptoms come and go. A few months ill, a few weeks well, then once again ill. Joints may be red and inflamed on the day the patient calls for an appointment. Today they are normal. There was fever a few days ago. Now it has gone. Last week a rash, this week none. Maybe the first symptom, a transient stomach pain, or a swollen gland, happened months ago. Unnoted then, recalled today, was that symptom part of the same disease process or was it something unimportant that can now be ignored? At the beginning of an illness laboratory tests may not inform.

One symptom suggests one diagnosis—Amirah's blurred vision—so a treatment is offered. A different symptom—weakness on one side—a different diagnosis, a different treatment. Then a decision is made and a treatment prescribed. One patient responds brilliantly. Another, whose symptoms seem identical, does not respond at all, or worsens. Flares, remissions, the illness never fully disappears. Patients ask questions but receive no sure answers.

This is the world of chronic disease.

In the world of acute illness, doctors order a blood test or an X-ray, give an antibiotic, an antidepressant, or a water pill, or perform surgery. The problem abates. Patient and doctor move on to other things.

For chronic illness, doctors do tests that may, but often do not, provide an answer. They try one medication after another, inching upward in sequence of strength and toxicity. Treatments alleviate inflammation or pain, slow an illness's progress, or induce a remission, but the remission lasts or it may not. Some treatments are tactics to prevent disability. Treatments do not cure chronic illness—the illness would not be chronic if they did. Physicians who treat patients with chronic illnesses accept uncertainty. It is part of the job.

Chronic illness frustrates many doctors, so they pass the patient on to someone else. "It's not something I can treat. Go to a specialist," they advise. Others, confused by waxing and waning or overlapping or unclear symptoms, attribute what they do not understand to a patient's neurosis. Others continue to climb the diagnostic tree, thinking that no matter how high they climb there will be still more branches. Then, at the division of some high branch they find there are *no* answers on both sides, nothing is *yes*, and so these doctors request just one more test, hoping that it at last will provide a name, an unending quest that may do more harm than good.

Everybody (doctors and journalists, that is) reads The New England Journal of Medicine, the well-known and widely quoted medical journal. As an entertainment bonus for its readers, the NEJM publishes a weekly puzzle, a medical mystery called a CPC, for Clinico-Pathological Conference.[4] CPCs report conferences, held at the Massachusetts General Hospital in Boston, the MGH, about difficult-to-diagnose patients. Each begins with a case description, follows with an expert's discussion and proposed diagnosis (the expert has not previously seen the patient), and concludes with a pathologist's answer that is confirmed by a definitive laboratory test, biopsy, or autopsy. CPCs are fun for doctors to read. Test

---

[4] Clinico- means what the treating doctors see in patient examination and laboratory tests. Pathology means what a laboratory test, biopsy or autopsy shows.

my brain against yours. No ambiguity. At the end, an answer—a diagnosis.

The case published on December 19, 2013, was that of a patient who had a rash for more than one and one-half years. She had been treated at two other hospitals and was now a patient at the MGH. She had seen many doctors and had had many biopsies to define the rash. The biopsies, done at different times by different doctors, had suggested several diagnoses, each of which has a different long Latin name. (Dermatologists revel in such names.) At the end of the CPC the pathologist announced one more such name. The Aha! moment. A definitive answer now!

But for this: Throughout this woman's ordeal, the blood tests always suggested—but failed to confirm—a type of lupus. And this: The best treatment for each of the different diagnoses, with the different Latin names, is the same. And one final thing: The different diagnoses are each so rare that there are no treatment guidelines for any of the rashes, just best guesses of what might work, hunches and "Let's try this now" treatment trials.

Each of the biopsies showed an interesting but somewhat different biology, the different biologies being the main teaching point and the reason for publishing the case as a CPC. The biopsies showed that the patient sequentially made an abnormal antibody first to one skin protein then to a second, then to a third. Each antibody in turn had sustained the rash, which continued to look the same, but each new antibody led to a different diagnosis and a different name. The process—an abnormal antibody irritated the skin and thus caused a rash—had been the same from beginning to end. Only the details—which skin protein was under attack today—had changed.

The patient may have had a different point of view. (I am guessing here.) To her, it was probably one horrible rash all along. I don't care about the name, she may have thought. Just get rid of the rash.

Nineteen months of the patient's life, to reach the Aha! moment—a final name—when no new treatment depended on that name. Her doctors then prescribed the only appropriate treatment at hand, something they could have done one and a half years before.

How does one teach this lesson—that "hard" data are not sacred? That one can accept ambiguity? Is it wrong to tell patients, students, and other doctors that we still see illnesses we can neither name nor understand?

We can say, "We do know a great deal; one fact will lead to another; we will understand more; and treatments will improve." We can teach that though there will always be mysteries, mysteries are not themselves bad, because they lead to better questions that, at some future time, will lead to better answers. Those who follow in our footsteps, perhaps these very students, will be better doctors then.

We can articulate the fact of uncertainty. We can break it into small, manageable pieces. We can identify elements of complexity. We can ask our questions within the context of Time. We can distinguish between process and cause. We can give weights to patients' individual choices. We can establish a dialogue between patient and doctor about what is and what is not known.

But, first, we need to know the boundaries of uncertainty.

Part II. The Boundaries of Uncertainty

7. Doctors Disagree

A recent unexpected email brought suddenly to mind memories that went back forty years. It came from Patricia, a former patient, one of my very first. I had been her doctor for about five years, then she had moved away.

Here are the memories: A young, pretty woman (the patient), her boyfriend, his ponytail, her parents, and her identical twin sister, who was not ill; the research studies we had done because she was a twin; her father fainting as he watched me draw his daughter's blood; her wedding in a beautiful colonial inn in a small New England town near our home; and a telephone call.

This is how the story begins.

Late on a sunny summer afternoon in my hospital, I replied to an overhead voice page: "Dr. C, call operator, stat."[5]

The page message was for my supervisor, but he was away and I had been assigned to take his calls. I called the operator back immediately, stat, we

---

[5] From Latin, *statim*, which means immediately.

say. She told me that a doctor from England was on the line, and she transferred the call to me.

The British caller, whom I did not know, began with an extended apology for interrupting my day. Patricia, he said when he, at long last, got to the point, is a young American woman who had recently been in London for a family wedding. A few weeks before her trip, at her college in America, she had volunteered to donate blood, but her donation had been refused because preliminary testing showed an antibody that coated the surface of her red blood cells and that made them unsuitable for use. Patricia had felt perfectly well, in fact well enough to volunteer to donate blood. The abnormal finding had been a surprise.

Because the trip to England was about to begin, and because she had family contacts with good information, she chose to consult the world's expert on that antibody, a doctor who worked in London. Seeing her, the doctor said the cause of the antibody was lupus. He advised her to return immediately to America to begin an exotic, even dangerous, treatment which, he said, we would provide.[6] He had sent relevant information to us by surface mail (one or two weeks by boat, no faxes or emails in those days), telling Patricia and her family to return home to await our call.

---

[6] We had ongoing contacts with his medical department; a former colleague of ours now worked with the British doctor who called.

They took the next flight back and now sat waiting. As the mail from England had not yet arrived, we knew nothing of what had transpired. Frustrated and anxious, Patricia's father telephoned the London doctor and paid for the call that I now answered. The Brits found this all very extravagant. Long distance! Trans-Atlantic! Could the family not have waited another week or two?

No, it seems, they could not.

When I saw Patricia a few days later, I agreed with the British doctor's diagnosis, but not with his treatment plan. She really was quite well. In fact, I said, I felt there was no need (at this time) to treat her at all. It was a not terribly important blood test abnormality that had been found. All we had to do was observe. My supervisor, one of the world's experts in this problem, when he returned concurred.

And that is what we did: Watch, with no treatment, over the next five years, at which time Patricia married and moved to another state.

Now, decades later, for irrelevant reasons, she found me and reached out by email. She wrote to me about the day that she and I first met. "I guess we were both so young," she wrote, "—it was fun. Also I don't know if I ever shared this with you (who can remember now?) but they put fear in me in England. Saying I would not live to see 30 and that the intervening years would be filled with illness and hospitalizations. So your reassuring, friendly manner was so important to me, trying to figure out life with [lupus]."

She was about twenty then. Today she is about sixty-five. She is generally well, but she did start treatment, of a mild and conventional, not exotic, sort, a decade or two after she had left my care.

The point is not that I was right and the Brits were wrong. The point is that different—even expert—doctors can see the same evidence and disagree. The center she had consulted in London was well known for lupus, as was ours. That does not mean that, faced with the same problems, we invariably made the same decisions. Despite the fact she was well, the British doctors interpreted her blood tests to show a very ill young woman. To me the same history and blood tests showed a well woman with an incidental abnormal antibody.

When even experienced doctors have such startling differences of opinion, how can we claim certainty? How can we say to a patient, "Here is what you *must* do"? Disagreement among physicians is well known to patients who have a chronic disease, as it is to their doctors. It is not so well known to the public at large.

* * * * *

The doctors in my hospital's division provide rheumatic disease consultation to inpatients in our three hospitals. Every Thursday morning we, trainees and senior physicians, meet to discuss the difficult consultations seen that week.[7] The point of the meeting is to teach. At our weekly conference, the junior physicians present the most challenging cases, then we discuss together what to do. We all learn.

Mostly we argue. (We are New Yorkers, after all.) "This part of the history needs more information," one doctor will say. "That point is irrelevant, a distraction, unimportant. This laboratory test should (or should not) be done," another will respond. "You should (or should not) give this medication. You should (or should not) treat at all." Someone cites a recent paper. Another recalls a similar case. We argue, but eventually we decide on a plan. The decision, never unanimous, is close enough to consensus to suffice.

Doctors rarely talk in public about physician disagreement—except to say (often in a court of law) that someone else is wrong. We rarely discuss the reasons we disagree: The science

---

[7] Of course we see all patients—and make treatment decisions—immediately when we are called. One point of the weekly review is be certain that all present agree that we did everything right, or, if not, to understand and correct what we might have done better.

is uncertain. The disease is not following the textbook's rules. At this moment, we really do not know.

Yet patients often must choose among doctors who disagree and who offer different treatment plans. Patients have the opportunity (or duty, or need) to choose among options. If given enough information to distinguish that which is certain from that which is a best guess, a patient can make her preferences known. She can negotiate with her doctors the choice that is best for her.

8. To Accept, or not To Accept, Uncertainty

Not everyone lives easily with uncertainty.

Let me tell you about Claudia. A girl. A woman. Which word I use is unimportant. The point is that in her early twenties, girl or woman, her life was at a bad place. Witty, sardonic, intelligent, articulate, Claudia was wise for her years, because, I suppose, she had been ill for nearly a decade.

She had very unusual symptoms and had seen many doctors. Her symptoms were so bizarre, and so seemingly unconnected, that each doctor had used a different diagnosis name. Her unusual combination of symptoms was so unlike anything that medical school teaches that some doctors accused her of faking it all.

At age sixteen her eyes became inflamed. The inflammation blocked the passage through which tears normally flow, then her retina tore and she underwent surgery on her eyes, first to open the pathway for the tears, then to repair the retina, then more surgeries to improve imperfect results, and still more surgery to make her eyes look normal again. Between surgeries a magnetic resonance imaging (MRI) scan, done to examine the nerves to her eyes, showed strange white patches on her brain. Some doctors thought those patches meant she also had multiple sclerosis; others disagreed. By the time I met her she had developed skin rashes and body pains. Many blood tests did not point to a single diagnosis, or they suggested many. Every doctor she saw was confused.

The abnormalities in Claudia's brain suggested multiple sclerosis. Some features of her rash suggested dermatomyositis, an uncommon rheumatic disease, and the reason she consulted with me. I did not think she had that diagnosis, but I did think that an available, if exotic, treatment officially approved for dermatomyositis might work for the brain and for the eye disease as well. The treatment is expensive; it required her insurer's approval. When I first applied to use that treatment, I was honest about the ambiguity of the diagnosis. The insurer said no.

Claudia and I appealed the decision. In our appeal, this time I was more imaginative; dishonest would not be untrue. I gave great emphasis to the existence of the rash and joints (both symptoms consistent with dermatomyositis) and barely mentioned the eyes, and brain (which were inconsistent). What I wrote was all true, just incomplete, with emphasis on the wrong parts. Thus did we win the appeal.

The treatment was a big commitment. Claudia received intravenous infusions for four consecutive days every month, each taking about four hours. She suffered distressing new symptoms during and for a few days after each infusion. It did not help that each session cost several thousand dollars.

The treatment did work. Her symptoms, once rapidly progressing, stabilized, or perhaps worsened at a slower speed. (Does one celebrate this kind of success when a patient is so young?)

There was a young man in her life. He left. Her eyes became inflamed again. The ophthalmologist told her that more surgery would be required. I don't know all the details from this point on. I have only the outline of the story now.

There was an argument at home, I am told, perhaps abetted by alcohol or drugs, or maybe not; I do not know. None of that is important now. At the beginning of her twenty-seventh year, this girl, or woman, it doesn't matter now, on a warm October night, fell, or perhaps jumped, from a high balcony, and died violently on the pavement below.

Suicide? Accident? I do not know.

An unexplained illness that recurred. A boyfriend who left. An argument. A balcony, a fall, and a death. Those are the facts I do know.

She died, I suppose, because she could not live with uncertainty, or perhaps because her view of certainty was more grim than had been mine. She died, I suppose, because I had failed to teach her a different way.

9.   Limits

I had finished the last draft—well, let me be honest, maybe the 15th draft—of this book. In fact I had begun to think that the book was done, when I received an email that challenged my thesis. Is it enough, the email made me ask, to teach patients and students to accept uncertainty? Do I not need to offer a solution as well?

This is what Laura's email said:

"I guess this is what the end of the road looks like."

This single line, so depressing, from someone so evidently depressed, caught me by surprise. Not because I did not know that Laura was depressed. I have practiced medicine for many years. I have seen many patients with chronic disease and I can recognize depression when it occurs. I also knew that Laura had reasons to be depressed.

No, I was surprised because I thought Laura was different. She is— was?—emotionally very strong, intellectually powerful, a leader in her field, very much and at all times in control, both of herself and of her complex professional world.

Of course I knew she was ill. Of course I knew we were running out of ideas to make her well. Of course I knew we had not made measurable progress for some time. But she and I had faced this level of frustration before and had found ways to overcome.

I had not anticipated her surrender, at least not now. Laura is action-oriented, private with her feelings, but not evasive. She is blunt, to the point, and concise. She has little patience with ambiguity. This is what I want to do, she would say. She had just taken a major step forward, on her own initiative, to improve her life.

Highly skilled in a challenging field, having just begun a demanding new job, she fell ill. Her confusing symptoms led different doctors to different conclusions. To whatever I attributed the cause, for whatever disease process I offered treatment, her most important symptom was incapacitating, widespread pain. Part of the mystery was that the source of the pain was unclear. Perhaps the pain came from her joints, or maybe from her muscles, or from her nerves. Pain that is intense and diffuse is hard to pin down. There were strong hints that the problem was autoimmune.

Her first doctors thought that an antibiotic had triggered an unusual reaction. She stopped the antibiotic but the pain stayed on. One doctor did electrical studies of her nerves, the kind in which the examiner inserts needles under the skin and administers electrical shocks to see how effectively the nerves transmit the sensation of pain. In those days, Laura had a sense of the ridiculous. "Now I understand the problem of Abu Ghraib," she said. "I thought torture had been outlawed."

At one point Laura consulted a national center that specializes in mysterious diseases. Not finding a cause, three different consultants from the center, in turn, advised: "Live with the pain," "Let's wait to see what ensues," and "Sometimes the best treatment is no treatment." The advice was unacceptable to her. The pain remained.

When she returned, we tried different treatments used for other autoimmune diseases, one after another. They did not work. We experimented with different pain medication regimens, which helped to a degree, but she found herself too groggy to perform her job. Though normally the national center offered patients only one visit to make a diagnosis, through personal contacts and persistence she secured an appointment to see a different group of physicians there, who might have different ideas. It was that second visit that occasioned her email to me. She wrote:

"I just received [my medical records from that visit] today. Please find the notes enclosed. I look forward to your take on their impressions. From my perspective, the neurology consult had more concrete recommendations. In contrast, the rheumatology consult really provided no direction nor real recommendations."

And then the devastating last line:

"I guess this is what the end of the road looks like."

And so she made me understand: It is not sufficient to discuss, or accept, uncertainty when a patient's problem is untreatable pain. Recognizing uncertainty does reduce frustration. It does (perhaps) justify watch-and-wait strategies. It does help a patient adjust to disability. But it does not ameliorate pain.

Her e-mail alarmed me. I immediately wrote back, offered to seek additional consultations, consider alternative medicines, or try (despite her and my own reluctance) antidepressant drugs. I asked if she had any further ideas herself, if she wanted to suggest or say something that we had not yet discussed, what she would do if she were in my place, or if she preferred that I dictate the next steps to her. (That last strategy works for people who have little knowledge of how limited medicine can be. I did not think it would work for her.)

Usually she responded quickly to my emails. This time she did not reply for a month, and then only because I wrote again, asking (as a pretext) that she validate a likely spam email I had just received that purportedly had come from her.

She answered: Yes, her email account had indeed been hacked, she said. Then she answered the question I had asked:

"I am not doing well. And nothing is happening. I will respond in more detail shortly."

Another month has passed. She has written nothing more.

This is the brick wall.

As I write about this today, the problem remains unresolved. I meant what I wrote to her. I am waiting for her reply. I do not want to give up. I pray that she will not surrender to the pain. My intention to help is clear.

But it is not enough, and intentions do not relieve pain. She said that she no longer wants to experiment with new treatments. I can offer her nothing new, except to try to maintain hope and to remain a friend. There are times to accept that our twenty-first century science is insufficient to the need. Absent hope, I can try to palliate, which means surrender and try no more. I do not think Laura and I are at this point yet.

Palliation of chronic, non-lethal illness differs from that offered to patients with advanced cancer or dementia. In the former the goal is to ease oncoming death; in the latter, to maintain dignity and happiness for one who can no longer understand. But when intelligence is intact and death not near, one palliates the emotion that accompanies loss of independence. It is easy to forget that sometimes one also needs to palliate inexorable, unremitting pain.

In the world of chronic illness, the patient soon enough understands that what is now is what will remain, that today's pain, or disability, or lack of independence, will continue for the next decade. Or two. Or three.

Sometimes the patient assumes command, becomes an advocate for self or class, forms or joins a self-help group, contributes to Internet blogs, or takes other actions that are positive for herself and for others like her. Sometimes the patient becomes passive, immobilized, accepting. Sometimes she withdraws. I suspect this is what is happening to Laura now. Unrelieved physical or psychic pain leads to this.

How can the doctor respond? It is useless to offer false hope or to lie. Disabled patients know full well what their futures will be. Tell a middle-aged paraplegic or someone whose joints are beyond surgical repair that they will be much better one day, and they will think you naïve and disbelieve your deceit. False encouragement makes the patient feel worse.

Being "there" for the patient, helping her feel not alone, helping her focus on things she can still do—this is my next role. Family and friends and doctors can offer methods for coping and suggestions or assistance to make the most of what function and strength remain. A person who has no use of her hands can still dictate a letter or a book or a legal brief. A person in a wheelchair can instruct and love a child.

Here is what I promised Laura. I will periodically reach out to you. I hope your discouragement will not prove dangerous. I pray that the inner strength I know you have will reassert itself. I will continue to look for new answers. I will not abandon you. I will figuratively hold your hand, and I will try in the ways I know to relieve your pain.

You said to me, "I guess this is what the end of the road looks like," but you do not need a road to continue on. The road seems closed just for this moment. There are moments still to come; you can use any imaginable means to bypass that which seems to stand in your way. This road may end, but you don't need a road to cross a field. You can still find another world beyond if you try.

Part III. Time

10. Measures of Time

We measure Time on many scales. Days, months, and years—the natural intervals in which humans live and that they instinctively know. Minutes, hours, decades, centuries, millennia—these are calculated, intellectual scales not intuited by man.

When I talk of medical things I prefer a more natural scale. I talk to my patients and my students about instant, clock, calendar, and generational time, the intervals in which medical events take place.

A patient suffers a seizure or fractures a leg: The event occurs in *instant* time. The diagnosis and treatment take place immediately. We soon know the outcome. The seizure ends, the leg is set. Accidents, ambulance calls, and medical decisions in television drama occur in instant time.

Fever and pain take place in *clock* time, hours and days. Within clock time we reflect and ask questions. Does the fever come and go? Does it occur once or twice a day? Did it start suddenly or slowly? Did it steadily grow in intensity, or does it wax and wane?

In clock time, the doctor can do blood tests, look at X-rays, consider the results, begin treatment, and look for improvement over the ensuing hours or days. The fever abates, the cough subsides, the blood count improves. In clock time the diagnosis and the outcome become clear. A treatment works or it does not. Everyone has experienced a medical event in clock time. No uncertainty here.

Illness that takes place in *calendar* time is less familiar to the world. Symptoms and recovery play out in months, and they come and go. Last month I was very ill, this month not so much. This month I have more good days and fewer bad ones. The bad days are no longer severe. Am I still ill? Will the pain disappear as it came?

In calendar time the patient makes an appointment to consult a doctor, but on the day of the visit there may be nothing to see. Joints once swollen are no longer so. The rash that came at the beginning is now gone. Blood tests, once startlingly awry, are no longer quite as bad, or changed in an unpredictable way. Then symptoms recur. And so it goes, off and on, until a pattern becomes clear. When effective treatment starts, relief is slow to come. The uncertain pattern reverses. A little better one day, not so the next. But in a few weeks, as the treatment takes effect, the bad days are fewer, the good ones more frequent, and remission seems possible. The outcome may not be clear for months. Calendar time is the visible scale of chronic disease.

Generational time is the least visible scale. A decade from now will today's teen-aged patient be able to carry or father a child? Will she see a normal middle age? Will she be disabled? If she is, will it be because of her disease or because its treatment damaged her muscles or bones, her heart or her brain? In chronic illness, disability occurs in generational time.

We know how to measure outcomes of medical events that take place in instant time. Blink and the event is done, the result known. The patient did or did not recover, did or did not die.

We also know well the outcomes of illnesses that take place in clock and in calendar time. Establish the diagnosis, do a trial or test a treatment, and measure the results after a few months or a year. Clinical research and most treatment courses take place in clock time. For much of clinical medicine, instant, clock, and calendar time decisions work well. No further thought is needed.

In chronic illness, improvement or worsening occurs in generational time, a time scale hard for both the patient and doctor to comprehend. If a patient improves six or twelve months after treatment begins, does improvement in that brief period of time say anything important about what the next twenty years will bring? In chronic illness, symptoms vary but rarely disappear. Damage may accrue even while the patient feels well.

In an acute illness the answer to a treatment trial is usually a clear *yes* or *no*, the treatment succeeded or it failed. The pneumonia, once here, is now gone. For a chronic illness that has no cure, whether the result is successful or not may remain unknown until the passing of extended calendar or even generational time. The answer to a treatment trial is not good enough if you report the patient's outcome after six, twelve, or twenty-four months, because the important question is the patient's state after six, twelve, or twenty-four years. Instead, one takes the proportion of patients who improve in a short time, or a measure of how much they improved, as a proxy for what will happen in the longer term. One may ask: Did the patient improve by 30% in the first year? Did the rate of worsening slow? In some cases, this depressing question may be the only way to measure success: Will fewer people be disabled or dead a generation from now?

Illnesses like lupus, Milagros' first diagnosis, attack many of the body's organs. Symptoms in the kidney may come at the beginning, after years, or never. Kidney symptoms, once begun, may or may not improve. The same applies to symptoms of the skin or the joints or the brain. Often, with successful treatment, symptoms in all the organs improve together, but sometimes the kidneys get better as the skin gets worse, leading to this conundrum: Did the treatment work (kidneys), or did it not (skin)? If the kidneys worsen, is it because the disease is still active, or because high blood pressure is damaging the kidneys in a different way, or because the inflammation is gone but scar tissue has formed? The answers can be very unclear.

You have treated the patient for several years. Today her kidneys have begun to fail. Some time ago I saw a young woman who first fell ill at age nine. Now she is in her forties and is facing kidney transplantation. Should we score this a success, since her kidneys functioned well for more than three decades, or not, since her kidneys have failed? The arthritis patient still walks, but she has had surgery to replace her knees—twenty years after her illness began. Is that success because the medication you prescribed kept her walking for two decades, or was it failure, that a surgeon was able to reverse?

How do you predict the outcome that will arrive a generation from now, when everything in medicine will have changed? Do you predict from what you know about those who were ill a generation past, when the drugs, surgical procedures, and other technologies were from a medical antediluvian age, when what you thought to be elegant treatment two decades ago is risible today? Will the fact that you prided yourself that you were able to postpone disability be ridiculed by the doctors of the next generation, who can prevent or completely cure?

Today we call lifelong treatment with a dangerous drug success, as we do with diabetes, epilepsy, and HIV. Tomorrow we may be able to cure the illness in a month, even predict and prevent its attack. How do you design a treatment trial the results of which will be judged a generation hence, when we will have new drugs, new tests, new machines, and probably new disease names? Can we do treatment trials that consider long-term outcome when, if we start that trial today, we may not even know who the patients are in twenty or thirty years. They may have moved away, their doctors may have retired or died, the rules for making their diagnoses may have changed, the records may use such different concepts that today's terminology is irrelevant or uninterpretable to future doctors, or the data may have been recorded in ways so foreign to today's thinking that the data that might answer the question cannot be found.[8]

Finally, what kind of criteria will we use to claim success? In rheumatoid arthritis, before joint replacement surgery arrived in the 1960s, and new magical biologic drugs came in the 1990s, disability was nearly guaranteed, the only question being how long it could be delayed. Today disability rarely occurs, but the disease lingers on. In the next generation, perhaps there will be a *bona fide* cure. Which will be the right measure: Delayed disability, no disability but continued medications, or cure? Success is a relative term.

It is not impossible to predict the long term. Diseases in animals give clues, imperfect though they may be, about how a disease will progress in humans. Short-term proxies—a bone density test, a cholesterol level—do predict future risk for fracture or heart attack. Perhaps, if a patient's arthritis goes into remission within the first year of treatment, the fact of remission will predict that she will be well in thirty years. Or perhaps not. Long-term prediction is just a guess, not more.

---

[8] The question is hypothetical. Some countries, Sweden, for instance for all health measures, and in some cases, like France for specific illnesses, have national registers that are structured to follow patients for decades; the United States has a few studies, such as the Framingham Heart Study, that do or have done similar things.

The best we can do is measure outcomes for clock and calendar times. So long as we manage conditions and not cure we may never know how to predict a person's health for generational time.

In chronic illness, doctors and patients live and make decisions simultaneously in instant, clock, calendar, and generational time. For you, the patient standing before me today, I can use this drug. It will reduce today's pain, but it will do you immense harm if you continue to take it for the next twenty years. Another drug will give less relief but does not cause long-term harm. Doctors and patients must negotiate the priorities of each other, for each time frame. Which do you prefer? Fast relief today (instant, clock), bad side effects later (calendar, generational), or less relief now, better outcome at twenty years? If the patient's and doctor's priorities are not aligned, will the patient disagree and go to another doctor? What if that other doctor is personable but a charlatan or a fool, and you fear he will do your patient harm?

There is no best choice among these different time scales. We consider them together, negotiating patients' and doctors' priorities or something in between. We cannot use a set of formal rules.

11. Heroes

On a warm, pleasant late September night, the doctors, nurses, and social workers at our hospital celebrated our heroes.

Who are they? They are our patients. They are those who, by their personalities, questions, and volunteered blood and time, give more to us and to other patients than they will ever receive. They are people whom we have grown to love as we cared for them for years.

I met Henrietta when she was eighteen. I saw her last when she was forty-nine.

Three decades ago, as I stood at the bedside of a very sick girl, I could not imagine her future. I could not predict the woman she would become nor could I predict how much I would grow to admire her. On that day long ago I saw only an extremely ill teenager, thrashing and moaning, near coma, with a disfiguring rash—a youngster, at the threshold of life, who might well die soon.

She survived that awful time. Though her recovery was marred by external and internal scars and by fragile bones, she grew to be a woman. Years later, now a joyful, instinctive teacher, she flaunted her scars before generations of medical students to teach them the damage that her illness could do, effusively praising those students who could identify the cause, laughing with and teasing those who were wrong. Over many years she volunteered gallons of her unusual blood for our studies.

Five feet four inches tall, 130 pounds, square of face and joyous of soul, this fast-talking, natural comedienne regaled us with awful jokes and atrocious puns, barely waiting for a response before moving on. She brought bags of mint candies to every clinic visit, handing one to each hospital nurse, receptionist, janitor, and me, requiring as payment that we listen to her worst pun for that day.

She spent many months in our hospital's beds. She endured surgeries to repair her bones and more surgeries to repair the repairs when the first ones failed. I lost count of her hospital admissions and operations. Stacked, her hospital charts (in the days in which we still had paper charts) were more than a foot high. Yet she mocked her fate and her pain. After her operations she marched up and down the clinic's halls, challenging medical students to analyze her gait, cheering aloud those who understood.

One year in a disease crisis her hair fell out and she became completely bald. Later, her hair began to regrow. At about that time she appeared in my office elegantly coiffed—a surprise, since, I thought, her hair could not have grown back so fast. Tactlessly, I asked, "Is that all yours?"

"You bet it is!" she declaimed, as, with a grandiose gesture and laugh, she ripped off her wig and waved it triumphantly above her stubble-covered but mostly still bald head. "I paid every cent!" she said.

Her rash had left large patches of pure white skin in place of its natural deep brown. "I have magic powers," she proclaimed to me. "I will make the color return." And it did, after many years, a victory she flaunted for the students, pointing out small dark specks in the remaining white that signaled the start of the pigment's return. When her hair really did come back, she grew a long braid, then marched about the room tugging on the braid and proclaiming, "I did it. I made my hair regrow." With jokes and puns, broad smiles and hearty laughs, she made us doctors feel good.

That first day at her bedside, I could not foresee my future hero, nor could I then know that she would become someone the entire hospital loved. What I did foresee was that the treatment that saved her life would in time destroy her bones. What I did not predict was how calmly she would accept the joint replacement surgeries that followed. Nor did I predict her deep involvement in her church, her future husband, or his love, so evident when he spoke her name on that warm September night in the ceremony that honored our heroes. I did not predict the strength with which she later accepted kidney failure, dialysis, and disfiguring cancer surgery the next year.

Then, thirty-one years after we first met, this once near-moribund child, now a vibrant wife and community presence, my hero, in a shower, changing a bandage that protected a plastic tube for dialysis that had been inserted into a large vein in her chest, she, by a slip of the scissors, accidentally cut the tube and bled to death, a senseless, horrific death that should never have been.

The nurses, the office staff, and the other doctors, and I, everyone who knew her, cried openly when we heard. Yet we smile, thinking of her, when we see her name on the plaque on the wall that honors our heroes. Henrietta is gone. The joy she gave endures.

We talk of diagnosis and treatment, but not about how passing time changes both a patient and a doctor. We do not talk about how a partnership evolves, how wariness turns into respect, how respect turns into trust, how the thoughts of one become the insight of the other, or how patient and doctor, doctor and patient, begin to make decisions as a team. We talk little of how a patient's trust in her doctor changes the tenor of the conversation. We never talk about how the doctor believes, trusts, respects, and begins to love his patient.

How does a doctor, standing at the bedside of a sick, near comatose child, foresee how much he will admire the woman she is to become, and how much she will enter his emotional life? How does he recognize the overwhelming power that her internal peace conveys, undimmed by serial hospitalizations and indescribable pain? How can he imagine the hero she will be? How can he imagine how much a small woman's outsize personality will invigorate so many lives?

12. The Arrow of Time

Everything we need to know is on the Internet.

When we doctors make our daily rounds, when we ask questions in our conferences, when we use an unfamiliar acronym, mention a rarely used drug, or describe a rash of a rare disease, out come the smart phones and tablets. In an instant an acronym's initials become a phrase, a drug's uses and toxicities are known, a rash is identified. On the Internet, everything is or can be quickly known.

Our science is so good, we know so much, how can we say that we do not know? We have such wonderful tools. We peer inside our bodies with MRI scans. We measure metabolism of organs and tumors with positron emission tomography (PET) scans. We use all sorts of micro-instruments and "minimally invasive" tests. We watch our thoughts with functional MRIs (fMRI). We multiply a single bacterium found in a patient a million-fold to identify and then destroy. We measure our genes, insert good ones in place of bad, create babies in test tubes, give mice human characteristics so that we can test our drugs, and transplant bone marrows and hearts and faces. So how is it possible that there are things that remain unknown? With such wonderful tools, when our science is so good, why is not every diagnosis certain? Why is not every cure secure?

Today science is very pleased with what it has accomplished. Such confidence—should I say arrogance?—is not new. Benjamin Rush proclaimed: "Our science has caught the spirit of the times and more improvements have been made in all its branches in the last twenty years than have been made in a century before." He said this in 1791![ii] In the early twentieth century a tuberculosis expert wrote of the treatment of Marie Duplessis, the Lady of the Camellias. "How distressing it is to read the prescriptions made in 1846," he said, then, with the wisdom of his day, concluded, "Only fresh air can help consumptives get well"[iiii]—four decades before streptomycin, the first successful antibiotic treatment for tuberculosis, entered the scene. Two centuries ago Beaumarchais mocked his fictional Dr. Bartolo, to the advantage of Mozart and Rossini, who highlighted Bartolo's pomposity in their Figaro operas. A century ago Flaubert ridiculed the self-assured assumptions of Madame Emma Bovary's physician husband. Today's doctors laugh at the self-assured errors of our teachers. Doctors fifty or one hundred years from now will surely laugh at what we believe to be truth today.

Today doctors do know a great deal. Tomorrow, we will know much more. Who can predict the future? Can you imagine that Wilhelm Röntgen, the early twentieth-century discoverer of X-rays, could have foreseen today's fMRI or PET scans? Could Willem Einthoven, inventing electrocardiograms, have envisioned coronary angiograms, bypass surgery, and heart transplants? Did Antonie van Leeuwenhoek, on first seeing microbes, think that one day there would be a microbiome,[9] or Gregor Mendel, with his colored peas, gene transplants?

From X-rays to fMRI, from cardiogram to transplant, these discoveries came one after the other in just an eyeblink of science's time. Since man first began to plant and harvest grain—was it 40,000 years ago?—since civilization began 10,000 years ago, we have known writing and science and one God for less than 5,000 of those years. Greco-Roman society thrived just 3,000 years ago. We have known microbes for only 400 years, Mozart for 200, and the genome for twenty. My parents did not know antibiotics for half their lives. My daughter has not heard of smallpox vaccinations. Today's

---

[9] The sum of all bodily bacteria, including those on the skin, mouth, intestine and elsewhere.

young adults do not know there once was a world without HIV. Only 500 years ago there was no Galileo; the best of medicine consisted of herbs, amputation, and drainage of pus. Five hundred years from now, in the year 2516, will today's high science seem as primitive to our followers as that of 1516 seems to us now?

When I was a new doctor we had just learned to monitor the heart rhythms of heart attack patients, and coronary care units were very new. The first antibiotics to treat *staphylococcus* and the first cancer chemotherapies had just arrived. Kidney transplants were a source of wonder. In those days I could not have predicted transplanting bone marrows, limbs, and faces. None of us could have imagined the arrival of HIV; targeted biologic therapies, today's wonder drugs, were beyond our ken. What will happen in just one or two decades that we are cannot imagine today? How arrogant is it to claim that we have little more to learn?

Time and knowledge move in one direction, the Arrow of Time. Today is a tiny moment, a dot, somewhere along the arrow's very long shaft, the length of which we do not know. Is today near the arrow's tail, which we also do not know, or close to its point? Ten millenia ago human beings began to settle in aggregate groups. Will civilization, will humanity, and with it the advance of science, exist for 10,000 years more?

Today's patient and many of her doctors assume that the fletching of the arrow's tail is very far behind and that the arrowhead, the acme of knowledge, is near. When the patient asks, "What will happen to me?" she expects a knowledgeable reply based on what we know today: "This (and nothing else) is your diagnosis. This is what the disease will do," followed by this additional reply, "This is the sure cure."[10]

If the question concerns only acute illness, the "sure cure" response might be true. A fracture heals. An appendix, once removed, causes no further pain. Of course, we can always do better. In acute medical events, a future doctor may be able to heal a fracture in an hour and cure pneumonia in half that time. All, not just some, of those who suffer a heart attack or stroke may someday survive.

Such certainty does not exist for chronic illness. For my patients, the arrow's head seems far distant. The origin of the knowledge base from which I work dates back only a past century or two and my most pertinent skills sometimes only a year or two. Sometimes from 19th century science and sometimes from that of the 21st century, I understand a little bit

---

[10] This discussion speaks to Western medicine, or medicine as it is practiced in the first world. In different cultures, and in which public health issues—infectious disease, malnutrition, civil strife—are more prevalent, such concerns as we discuss are irrelevant.

about how a patient's illness did its damage and how it might continue to cause more if I have no cure. I can guess what new things doctors may learn about this illness in the very near future. Yet I cannot begin to imagine what doctors will know decades from now, or how they will conceptualize, diagnose, or prevent or cure my patients' illnesses then.

Future doctors may be startled to see how we slow we were to see obvious clues that, lacking a technology soon to be invented, might have pointed to solutions of some of the mysteries we now face. Here are some examples from the recent past: Fractures of bones, weak because of poor nutrition, preventable once we understood the role of vitamin D; psychoses and dementias, attributed to personality, now recognized as structural brain disease because of CT scans, MRIs, and fMRIs; random bizarre infections completely incomprehensible until we understood HIV; duodenal ulcer, treated as anxiety and stomach acid production until we learned of the bacterium that starts and perpetuates the sore.

If future doctors are kind to us, they may excuse our ignorance if they understand that technology not then available, later invented, was required to bring the hidden to light. They may be sympathetic, knowing that without the new technology we could not possibly have understood. Or they may laugh at how oblivious we were.

I do not think that, today, we are anywhere near Time's Arrow's point. For my patients with chronic illnesses, I cannot answer their questions with unchallengeable facts, because what we know today can always be challenged, nor can I don the mask of certainty that, younger and more naïve, I may have once displayed.

Instead I say to them: This is what we know today, this is what we do not, and this is what we might know soon. It is not important that I give your disease a name. The name is only a label. To know the disease process, how it is affecting you, and how I can safely change that process, is what we need. I will comfortably use those tools that I understand and negotiate with you the possibilities when knowledge fails.

I will also tell my patient: Please do not demand certainty of me. If I do not doubt, I will not have an open mind. If I keep in mind what I do not know, I have freedom to explore. There is no place for arrogance in this plan. Time will pass, we will learn more, and things will change. I hope that my patient will agree.

13. To Teach These Lessons

Medical students mostly see patients who are in hospitals; they mostly learn about the acute medical events that led to the hospitalizations, like heart attacks, injuries, and flu. Patients who have chronic illnesses do get hospitalized, of course, and students do see them, in short slices of time, for treatment of acute complications, like pneumonia. Or they see them for brief office visits on clinic days, when the patient most often is stable. Exposed to chronic illness in this way, the medical student has little feeling for or incentive to explore the concerns of long-term management, or even the implications of what he or she has seen.

A student's time on a medical topic or specialty is short, one month, maybe two. Students rarely see how diseases evolve over time. They do not appreciate the emotion and adjustment as an ill person begins to understand and then adapt (or not) to illness or disability, or how one returns, often slowly and with terror, from an episode of near death to engage life again.

Concerned about what students do not see, I developed a medical school course to teach about chronic illness. The emphasis of the course was Time, spelled with capital T. I constructed the course as a seminar: A few patients, a few students, and me, talking around a table. On seminar days patients came from their jobs or other activities. They came, that is, from their non-ill lives. They wore street clothes, appeared as themselves, not undressed or in hospital gowns, not impersonal, abstracted from their lives and dissected for study, not, in T. S. Eliot's words,

formulated, sprawling on a pin,
...pinned and wriggling on the wall.[iv]

The patients I invited to the seminar all had chronic illnesses. Because I wanted to discuss how patients manage uncertainty, and also because I wanted the students to approach patients with open minds and not to parrot back textbook inanities, I made it a point to invite people whose illnesses were complex and not clearly labeled with diagnosis names. Several, like Claudia, who spoke at the seminar, had diagnoses that were very obscure.

I wanted these special people to describe the uncertainty in their lives, how they learned to deal with complicated and contradictory information, and how they did or did not manage to partner with their doctors in their medical care.

As I watched the seminars progress, in my mind the patients spoke brilliantly. They defined themselves by their appearances and by their occupations—student, writer, nutritionist, police officer, and more, not by their afflictions. They made it clear that their lives were not consumed with their illnesses—a point I had hoped they would display. Their intrinsic personalities were the important thing. To them, even those who had faced or were facing possible death, the names of their illnesses were not the major point. What mattered was the illnesses' power to disrupt their daily lives.

This is what we talked about: How do you adjust to being ill? How do you think about and plan for disability? Can doctors and patients plan for both the short and the long term simultaneously? What do doctors and patients *not* tell each other? How do you make choices when facts are ambiguous? What happens when doctors disagree? What are the effects of outside things, like family, culture, and insurers? How do you maintain ego strength when you are ill?

The patients taught, and the students learned, explicit answers to the questions. The students' essays at the end of the course showed they understood this: Chronic disease changes one's sense of personhood. Patients make choices concerning their own care, complying with or rejecting what their doctors prescribe. Ego strength is a patient's key to success. These are important lessons.

As the course ended, from the students' comments, I learned that what I had taught was incomplete. I thought I was teaching about Time and chronic illness, but I later understood that the larger lesson was about uncertainty itself, ever present, not easy to dismiss, a burden for both patients and doctors. Another lesson is that the doctor's job to identify and talk with his or her patient about uncertainty, to capture and control it, and to use it as a tool for a positive good.

I also learned that the students did not want to hear about uncertainty.

They were probably right. The students were in their first and second years of medical school, that is, they were beginners. They did not yet know enough basic facts, not even the names of the chronic diseases that afflicted the seminar patients. It was too early to teach this lesson, and so they were confused.

As, it seems, was I. How do you teach uncertainty to medical students when equanimity, confidence, and the appearance of being all-knowing is the rule? To whom and when do we need to teach that lesson? To the students? To the patients? Or am I wrong? Do I need to rethink what uncertainty means to me?

Part IV. The System's Rules

14. How True is Truth?

If you read medical school textbooks you will think that any doctor, hearing a patients symptoms, if he requests enough tests, can reach a correct diagnosis.

There is, of course, another "if". The doctor can make a diagnosis if she asks the right questions, understands the answers, sees both visible and hidden information, synthesizes all that information and puts it into the right context.

There are two more requirements: The doctor must begin the inquiry with an open mind. After having made a decision, the doctor must be prepared to rethink everything as new, possibly contradictory, information arrives.

When a patient comes to a hospital, someone, the first doctor or nurse to see him, assigns a tentative diagnosis. Every subsequent doctor, nurse, physician's assistant, or medical student enters the patient's room knowing that label. Where electronic charts are used—as they are in most American hospitals today—a doctor most often, to save time, begins a chart note by copying and pasting the note written before. Our own hospital allows—indeed prefers—that the doctor write a "structured" chart note. If the writer elects the structured-note option prior notes and laboratory findings automatically populate the new note that is about to begin. However, while it assures the readers and writers that past information is not lost, a structured note neither assures accuracy nor corrects error. It makes it difficult ever again to think of the patient as an unknown.

On the day a doctor first meets a patient, even if the patient's first words are impossibly vague ("I feel sick"), at the end of the encounter the doctor assigns a diagnosis and a code number from which all subsequent steps follow. In fact, contemporary electronic medical records do not allow recording of unclear diagnoses. If (to the doctor) the diagnosis is ambiguous, his response will be to do more tests. By convention and required structure every chart note ends with these three bullet points: Diagnosis, additional test plan, and treatment plan. In fact, it was because her chart notes were written in this structured format that I was able to record the thoughts of the six neurologists who saw Amirah over the Christmas holiday, as I described in chapter 5.

Sad to say, professors like me usually teach our students that correct diagnosis is the most important part of a patient encounter, and that all our decisions will depend on the diagnosis we have chosen, so we challenge young doctors to be precise. If a diagnosis seems unclear, we ask our students, "What additional tests can you do that will make it known?" We seldom teach, "We can make a better decision six weeks or six months from now than we can today. Leave it alone for the moment. You do not need such precision right now. It will not make a difference," or, "The problem is evolving. Keep the patient comfortable, anticipate problems, use conservative treatments to keep those problems controlled, but do not (yet) use the fashionable (also very dangerous) drugs. Leave yourself an escape route. Do nothing irreversible—at least not now."

We teach a different lesson: "Be compulsive. Keep testing. The more tests you do, the more likely you will find a diagnosis."

Though we call them facts, symptoms are very subjective, are described in different vocabularies, are suggestions to physicians that are subject to different interpretations by different observers at different times. Ask a patient, "Where is the pain?" "In my muscles," she replies, or "maybe here," as her hand wanders over her abdomen or an entire leg. Is that really information one can use? Ask, "What is the pain like?" The answer is descriptive and impossibly imprecise. What does "burning" or "deep" or "dull" actually mean? To the question,

"How long has it hurt?" is "Maybe a few weeks" or "Since about Easter" an answer at all?

If the patient's response comes in many forms, how individual doctors interpret that response comes in many more. A medical resident wrongly wrote in the chart—only I, who had the most experience in this field, saw the error—that the drug-caused blush on Amirah's cheeks was a lupus rash. Because doctors writing notes tend to refer to notes by others of their own training level or specialty interest, the error was repeated (copied and pasted) in each subsequent note by junior and non-specialist doctors and was included in the discharge summary (written by the most junior member of the team). In a different case, a senior physician, seeing my bed-bound patient admitted with pneumonia, and not seeing the severe arthritis that caused her to be bed-bound, ordered her to walk several times a day to speed her recovery. A cardiologist scolded a third patient of mine, a dwarf, four-and-one-half feet tall, for staying in bed when he should be exercising, then turned on her heel and left the room, oblivious to his plea that the bed was too high, that he had no stool or mechanical means of lowering the bed, and that he could not get down! For a fourth patient, an abnormal blood test, dutifully charted, suggested a serious clotting disorder to the admitting physician, but the test was abnormal because a medicine that changes the result had been given in the emergency room, evident elsewhere in the chart but not in the summary note the doctor upon which the doctor relied.

These are simple, stupid charting mistakes recorded as though they were facts and the only information other doctors needed to know, never corrected, perpetuated as relevant to the end of time.

If the patient's chart is the only source of information, Amirah had a rash, the arthritic patient and the very short man both refused to leave their beds, and the other patient had a clotting problem. Though I spoke to the doctors, the notes remain uncorrected, except in my protest notes, which were not cut and pasted and will likely not be read. I have neither the authority to correct the notes of others nor to dictate which notes they will paste into their own new notes. The person who later reads the chart will likely assume the prior notes to be true.

When thoughtfully obtained, interpreted, and recorded, the answers to core medical history questions are facts. When correct, physical examination observations do have value. But there is no way after the fact to prove that what was once written was correct or true. Insurers rely on these notes to pay a patient's diagnosis-based bills. Administrators praise or censure doctors for their adherence or non-adherence to diagnosis-based best practice rules. But if diagnosis depends on "facts" that might be wrong, why should precision diagnosis be our anchor? If treatment is offered, why should we base that treatment on a name rather than on the knowable, but uncoded, patient's symptoms and needs?

15. Binary Thinking

Two roads diverged in a yellow wood
...and I—
I took the one less traveled by
And that has made all the difference.[v]

Robert Frost

Administrators love the diagnostic tree. When everything is a *yes* or a *no*, every piece of paper that a doctor submits—to get approval for a test or treatment, to demonstrate competence, and to get paid—is easy to grade.[11] There are check sheets and treatment protocols and algorithms. There are always just two roads, a right choice or a wrong. The branches of the tree

---

[11] When I speak of payment or reimbursement, I do not refer to my personal income. If a test or medication already performed or administered is not (after the fact) approved, either the administering agency (hospital or clinic) or the patient will be asked to pay the bill. The physician who ordered the test or medication will likely receive a note of censure.

separate; they do not cross or merge. Each branch reaches a definable end.

In the paperwork of clinical practice, the branch points are called criteria, guidelines, and algorithms. We follow the *yes* or *no* roadmaps to establish diagnoses, judge an illness' severity, and make treatment decisions. Does the patient have fever, *yes* or *no*? If *yes*, your options are these. If *no*, the options are different. Do a blood count. Is the white blood cell count high? Another branch point, another *yes* or *no*. These are well traveled roads. They offer binary decisions, never hinting or believing that sometimes there is neither a *yes* nor a *no*.

Why do we use criteria, guidelines, and algorithms? To make the complex simple. How do we use them? To verify a suspected diagnosis, predict a prognosis, or set a treatment plan.

To use diagnostic criteria we often consult a published table or diagram that lists symptoms and results of laboratory tests. Next to every symptom there are check boxes, one for *yes*, another for *no*. Answer each question. Total the check marks. Enough *yes*es checked, the suspected diagnosis is correct; too many checked *no*, think of something else.

Often *diagnostic* criteria are used to enroll candidates in a research study, such as a drug treatment trial. The criteria include typical patients—reagent-grade patients, a friend of mine says—so that the answer to the trial will be clear. Trials exclude unusual patients because they might confuse the result.

There are other criteria for disease *severity*. If a patient has enough points, there is a need to change treatment, to enroll the patient in a trial, or to offer a prognosis. Score the number of points at each visit or twice a year; chart the points to show that the patient is better or worse. If all the points disappear, you can grade the treatment a success. Some doctors are now graded—and paid—according to how meticulously they maintain such charts or follow criteria sets published by others.

How well do criteria work? Fairly well, I suppose, if the patient has a typical illness.

However, the information criteria impart depends on the sort of person to whom the patient is compared. Criteria do not stand alone. If a patient has a symptom or laboratory finding of x, and someone who is normal—or someone who has a different disease, or a similar disease, does not, then x may be an appropriate criterion.

The comparison group one chooses depends on the question asked. The comparison group could be normal people, or it could be people with another illness. If the latter, that illness could be similar to the illness in question, or very different. Fever is a reasonable criterion to suspect influenza (or Ebola virus) in a group of people who one assumes are healthy, like a schoolroom class or a group of people waiting to board an airplane. Fever is not a good criterion for influenza (or Ebola) in children on a leukemia ward or in adults on a tuberculosis ward, because many would have fever caused by something else.

If the point is to distinguish between two diseases that look alike, such as rheumatoid arthritis and lupus, the criteria must be very narrow. Arthritis would be a good criterion for rheumatoid arthritis in a population of normal people but it would be a poor criterion to distinguish it from lupus in an arthritis clinic because arthritis occurs in similar ways in most patients with either disease. In the arthritis clinic, a blood test found only in patients with lupus, but not in those with rheumatoid arthritis, or *vice versa*, would be a better criterion.

Severity criteria help doctors decide which treatment to prescribe, or whether a treatment has worked. If a patient has arthritis, count the number of inflamed joints at the start of treatment. If the number is high enough, begin the treatment.

Count the joints again after a few weeks. If the number has gone down enough, you have reached the goal; the treatment continues. If the number has not gone down, or has gone up, it is time to declare the treatment a failure, to try something else.

Criteria seem to bring order to chaos. They outline a path to take. So how can one complain?

Well, what, exactly, are criteria? Who devises them? Who makes the lists? How do we know they are true?

Criteria, guidelines, and algorithms are the published deliberations of an appointed expert committee that chooses the *yes* or *no* questions and the total number of *yes*es and *no*es that will be used.[12] The committee defines the answer for each question. How high must a temperature be to call it fever? How swollen must a joint be to call it arthritis? Each element requires a *yes* or *no* answer. Perhaps a little bit swollen suffices for the *yes*, or perhaps it does not. The committee is free to decide.

---

[12] Criteria most often establish diagnosis, for instance, a combination of three of the following symptoms indicate X disease. Guidelines suggest steps to take to establish a diagnosis or to initiate a treatment change, for instance, after trying drug A, go on to drug B. Algorithms stratify guidelines into binary answers, for example, if M is true, do this; if M is not true, do that.

Criteria do not offer alternatives. If fever is the chosen criterion, you cannot substitute pulse rate instead. Criteria often require exclusions. Answer *yes* if the patient has the symptom but does not also have something else. For example, anemia can count for a lupus diagnosis only if you have proved that the anemia is not due to bleeding or to iron deficiency.

There are no criteria for criteria. Each committee decides for itself what to do.

Who chooses the members of a committee's panel? Sometimes government agencies choose them, sometimes diagnosis-focused interest groups, and sometimes professional groups.

There are no criteria for who sits on criteria committees. Sometimes they are experts who know the most about the problem, sometimes non-experts, such as general physicians (who will be the ones who use the criteria), sometimes patients, and sometimes non-physician scientists. Professional groups from different countries issue competing criteria. Approval and use of criteria are by consensus. There is no final body that says whose criteria will reign.

Expert panels have procedures to exclude bias. Sometimes their rules are so strict they exclude anyone who has ever offered an opinion—spoken publicly, written a paper—on the topic, the result being there is no true expert on the panel. That is not always a bad thing, because those bound by the rules will be mostly non-experts. Panels composed solely of experts, who know many potential sources of error, tend to issue rigid sets of criteria, most easily usable by other experts. Such criteria work well for clinical trials. Panels composed of non-experts tend to issue pragmatic but imprecise guidelines, usable by generalists. They work best to guide doctors in practice.

How do panels choose what elements of a diagnosis to include?

Sometimes they do this systematically. They first review everything that has been previously written on the topic, identify the strengths and weaknesses of what has gone before, and then agree on tentative rules—how abnormal must that blood test be? They then test the tentative rules with actual patients. If the test does not identify the right patients, the committee examines reasons why it may have failed, rewrites the criteria, and runs the test again. These types of criteria, very data-based and error-checked, are called "evidence-based".

Other committees rely on the opinions of experts, probably well-founded, but not checked against real patients. They are instead discussed and argued around a table. These types of rules are called (sardonically) "eminence-based".

Doctors, patients, news media, and the Internet regularly cite criteria. Patients tell me, "I know I have this disease. I looked it up on the Internet. I fit all the criteria." News broadcasts cite the results of treatment trials, not asking who fit the enrollment criteria for the tested disease or who was refused. Almost never does the reporter or broadcaster discuss who wrote the criteria, to whom were the comparisons made, or why the criteria exist at all. In fact, they rarely know that many sets of criteria exist for the same disease, let alone how they were devised. Reports that contradict one another abound.

Criteria do have an important role. They provide a degree of certainty regarding uncommon illnesses that an average practicing doctor may never have seen. They allow treatment trials to proceed. Criteria, at least those that are well done and consensus-based, do little harm and much good.

Perhaps. Or, perhaps, too intense belief in the power of criteria increases confusion when complexity holds sway.

16. Are Diagnosis Codes Lies?

Today the doctor's world is filled with code numbers, especially those called ICD (for International Classification of Diseases). There are code numbers for diagnoses, for procedures, and for severity of disease or injury. Doctors and hospitals must use these numbers in their chart notes, their requests for blood tests and X-rays, and their hospital discharge summaries, and bills. Documents lacking appropriate code numbers may be rejected. No code, wrong code: An MRI scan will not be done; a bill will not be paid. Most medical documents contain not one but many codes, one for the primary diagnosis, another for something else, say high blood pressure, or obesity, or headache, another for something else. The more codes, the more complex the case, the higher the bill.

Codes do not allow for uncertainty, permit ambiguity, or allow alternative paths. The ICD codes are very precise. Those used in the United States through September, 2015, consisted of five, sometimes six digits, sometimes letters, with a dot in the middle, in this format, 123.456. Those codes were those of the ninth version of the ICD, called ICD-9. ICD-9 lists 17,849 separate diagnosis codes.

Here are some examples: Pneumonia was code number 486 (if you did not know the infecting germ), or 480.0 through 480.9 if you knew that the germ was one of the most common ten. The code for diabetes was 250.00 or 250.01, or 250.02, depending on some details. Arthritis of the hip was 715, or 715.09 or 715.15, again depending on the type. You get the point: Many codes, more precision, easier for policy-makers to study, for billers to bill, or for payers to refuse to pay.

More precision? Although many illnesses are different in different races—lupus, for instance, is three times more prevalent, and two times more severe, in blacks compared to whites—there are no ICD subcodes for race, and none for sexual preference (except for psychiatric diagnoses and "high risk homosexual behavior"). So how precise can these codes be?

On October 1, 2015, the tenth version, ICD-10, came into use. The ICD-10 codes now number 141,742, almost ten times as many codes as before![vi] Did I say there was an obvious logic connecting the numbers of ICD-9 to those in ICD-10? I did not, because there is none that I can see.

Some of ICD-10's code numbers are incomprehensible. I recently looked up the ICD-10 code for protein in the urine (proteinuria). I found separate numbers for *unspecified proteinuria, isolated proteinuria, proteinuria cause unknown,* and *proteinuria other unspecified.* I have no idea what the difference among these different codes might be. At the bedside or in the clinic, such distinctions make no sense at all.

Andrew Pollack of the *New York Times* mocked ICD-10's pretense to precision[vii] by pointing this out: There is a unique code number for an injury sustained while jumping off burning water skis, another code for injury in a spacecraft, and a third code for injury by an orca whale.

Katie Bo Williams, writing in Healthcare Dive,[viii] listed what she called the 16 most absurd codes, including code numbers for being bitten by a pig, being injured in a swimming pool in a prison, being struck by a duck (which has a code number different from that of being struck by a macaw), and having a bizarre personal appearance. Ms. Williams' list also includes the water skis and the whale.

At lunch I shared this information (ranted, actually) with my brother, who is a biologist. He asked me a question, and I sought the answer. That is how I discovered that ICD-10 has a code number for injury by a bite of a black widow spider

(T63.31), which is different from the code number for a brown recluse spider's bite (T63.33). There are also sub-codes for the spiders. One can score whether the bite (by either black or brown spider) is an unintentional injury (T63.311 or T63.331), an intentional self-injury (T63.312 or T63.332), an assault-induced injury (T63.313 or T63.333), and an undetermined reason for the injury (T63.314 or T63.334). (Another point of uncertainty: Exactly how does one commit assault by spider? I suppose it can happen.)

Though the spiders look a bit alike—in fact the question arose as my brother and I tried to identify one hiding in a dark corner in my house—the distinction may make sense. Several days following a bite by each of the spiders the evolution and appearance of the wounds inflicted is different, the black widow's bite causing more general symptoms throughout the body, that of the brown recluse being more locally destructive, like an abscess. But the rule is that the code must be assigned when the patient seeks treatment, not at some future time. At that anxious moment in the emergency room (as one possibly stares at the squashed indeterminate remains of the animal spread on a dirty tissue), will either the doctor or the patient know or care which spider is which?

Want to do a laboratory test? The code must match the purpose of the test. If you want to do a chest X-ray for a person who has diabetes and who has fever and cough, the code for diabetes does not suffice to order the X-ray, but including it may increase the bill because the patient now has several diagnoses and is therefore more complicated to treat. To justify the chest X-ray you have to add a different code if the patient is short of breath, a different one if he has a cough, several different ones for pneumonia, depending on the part of the lung and the specific germ, or still another for asthma or for emphysema if either coexist. I have not yet mastered ICD-10.

The codes offer apparent precision, but one would be a fool to think them accurate. Doctors choose the code that will not be challenged and that will get the test done, not the code they believe is right. No one later amends, or even has the opportunity to amend, a code to say that the X-ray was negative, that the patient had bronchitis, not pneumonia, so was sent home, or (worse) that the film showed unsuspected cancer or rib fractures (suggesting domestic abuse).

Once assigned, code numbers do not admit any change at all. One assigns the codes at the time the patient is seen, not after the tests have returned and the final decision made. At best a billing agent at some future date will look at the chart to see if the doctor recorded the right things that justify the bill, indifferent to whether those things were or were not correct. There are no code numbers that allow the doctor to be honest—to say, "I think it's normal, but I want to be sure," or "This patient is sick, but I don't know quite why. Let's explore possible causes." In fact, if one did write such honest things, the test would be refused, or the bill would not be paid. At best, ICD-10 encourages doctors to shade the truth; at worst, it forces doctors to lie.

How valid are ICD codes? They work, more or less, for today's common or fashionable diagnoses. ICD-9 began in 1975. It was revised for ICD-10. What we think is a reasonable diagnosis can change. I have listed in an endnote[ix] things that are new in the last forty years. The list is incomplete. It consists of just the things I recalled in the last five minutes or so. How can we compare today's codes with those that were appropriate a generation ago?

Codes imply certainty. The problem is to believe that because you have assigned a code, you now know what the diagnosis is.

A few hours after she was born, doctors in the newborn nursery, conducting a routine examination of a newborn child, found that the ball of Deirdre's hip had slipped from its socket. This is a relatively common problem among newborns whose hip socket is too shallow. The diagnosis of a congenital hip dislocation is so common in fact that many state laws require that nurseries perform a simple physical examination maneuver to check every newborn child for this problem.

Deidre's doctors prescribed a body cast to be placed over her pelvis to hold the hip in place. She wore the cast for a few months until the hip socket deepened enough to be secure. A body cast is not the most pleasant thing one can do to a newborn baby (or to its parents), but not treating the loose hip would mean that Deirdre would have had a very bad limp for the rest of her life. The examination takes just a few seconds; to treat the dislocation involves a cast for a few months, a small price to pay. Deirdre grew to be a normal, athletic child.

Now in her late 20s and married, she felt pain in her knee, or maybe at the back of the leg, or maybe at the hip or sacroiliac (SI) joint. I am imprecise because she herself was unclear. Eventually a physical therapist suggested the pain came from inflammation at the SI joint. If that were so, it would be a sign of a rheumatic disease. Her doctor ordered an MRI scan, listing (for insurance pre-approval) the ICD-9 diagnosis code 720.9 for sacroiliitis, inflammation of the SI joint. Had he used the code 724.5, back pain not otherwise specified, approval to obtain an MRI would likely have been denied.

The radiologist who read the MRI saw that number.[13] His report said that Deirdre had a slight abnormality at the SI joint.

---

[13] I did not meet any of these people or talk to them. My comments are judgments I made based on the content of their notes.

I have seen reports like this before. Those who read MRIs try to answer the question asked and sometimes hedge their bets. The reader of the MRI more or less said this: "I do not really see the abnormality you expect me to see, but I know that is what you think, and so to be cautious, I will qualify my reading with a lot of extra words. Your patient may have just the slightest bit of an abnormality at the SI joint." To me, such a report says, "No."

Deirdre's doctor seems to have thought it said "Yes" because he prescribed a medicine appropriate for SI joint inflammation, indicated by published guidelines for treating sacroiliitis, but one that would be unwise for the pregnancy she planned. (The guidelines did not discuss possible pregnancy.) She sought another opinion, in which a different doctor suggested another guideline-directed medication that would also preclude pregnancy. That was the reason she came for a third opinion. Dissatisfied, Deirdre had asked a family friend, who spoke to a colleague of mine, who suggested she ask me. She wanted treatment, but she wanted to have a child as well.

She and her husband arrived with stacks of medical charts and pounds of X-ray films. My examination showed that Deirdre has very loose joints, not terribly unusual in someone with a history of hip dislocation at birth, not serious and not rare. People with loose joints are very flexible. They become the gymnasts and the ballerinas whom we applaud.

I looked at the MRI films they brought. I saw no signs of inflammation of the SI joints, just a little extra fluid. To be sure it was normal, (because reading MRIs is not one of my best skills) I asked our own hospital's radiologists to comment. They are experts in this field and they agreed with me. The extra fluid was because Deirdre had loose joints, something one does not treat with powerful drugs. Protect the joints, exercise in a careful way—was all she needed to do.

I am speculating, but I think this is what had happened. The code number on the MRI request misdirected the first radiologist, who, eager to please, wrote an ambiguous report. The doctor who had ordered the film had wanted to see his hunch proved right. He read the report, but did not himself look at the films. The next doctor had done the same. What each doctor saw in the films had been distorted by 720.9, a number that implied precision, which led to an error, followed by a chain of guideline-directed decisions that were wrong.

The code numbers justified payment for Deirdre's MRI scan, because the only questions asked are whether the rules have been followed, not whether the diagnosis is correct. Armed with the MRI report, her doctors adhered to the best practice guidelines written for 720.9 and wrote the appropriate prescriptions. In fact, because the doctors all used 720.9, had they not prescribed the treatments they did, they might have been faulted for poor practice.

Prescribe a treatment not sanctified by guidelines for that code? Is the treatment you prescribe the only one appropriate for this particular patient, even though the patient does not fit guidelines or is looking forward to pregnancy? Too bad. The insurer may refuse to pay. An administrator might censure the doctor for improper care. The doctor may be sued. There are people whose job is to find and punish doctors who do not follow best-practice guidelines.

The intent is good; guidelines do help prevent bad practice. But when the diagnosis is ambiguous, or when the code does not precisely fit, or is even outright wrong, following guidelines rigidly may create bad practice instead.

Guidelines do not allow a physician to admit that she has sixty percent confidence that her diagnosis is correct. Treatment algorithms do not answer what might be the best thing to do when there is only twenty percent chance that a patient has a diagnosis that might be cured by your treatment and very little chance that a patient with a different diagnosis will be harmed. What if the chance is seventy percent that the diagnosis is right, but fifty percent that, if you prescribe the preferred treatment and the patient has a different diagnosis, the patient will be harmed?

Treatment guidelines are easy to find. On most hospital computers, in the office, or on the Internet, type in the ICD code, 9 or 10, and guidelines for its diagnosis or treatment will appear on your screen. You are expected to follow what the computer tells you to do. In fact, in many hospitals and pharmacies, computer programs will prevent a doctor from entering an order not sanctioned by the assigned ICD code. These programs prevent stupid mistakes, which is good. They hinder necessary treatment when the patient does not match the entered code, which is bad.

Diagnoses, guidelines, codes, and algorithms are all man-made. For any single patient there may be no correct code. For reasons of convenience or efficiency a doctor may assign a wrong code. A patient has symptoms of several diseases: Choose the code that will get the test done or the prescription filled. Ignore the code that will tempt a bureaucrat to issue a hold. ICD-10's 141,742 codes will not resolve that ambiguity. One cannot assign a truthful code to what one does not understand.

The summer she turned 15, Shoshana traveled to Israel to work at a kibbutz. She returned home with abdominal cramps and diarrhea. Numerous tests by her pediatrician did not explain why she was ill. A gastroenterologist did a screening test for lupus, I do not know why, since her symptoms did not suggest this disease.

The screening test for lupus was positive. Follow-up confirming tests were negative. We call that kind of result a false positive, a not terribly uncommon event. This is the interpretation: Positive screening test, negative confirming test—lupus is not the problem. Nonetheless, the positive screening test was the reason Shoshana's parents brought her to me.

I said: "No. Not lupus. It is better to look for more obvious things, Crohn's disease (a type of intestinal inflammation), let's say." Shoshana saw more doctors and did more tests. Sharing my thinking, one of those doctors prescribed high doses of corticosteroids ("steroids") to treat possible Crohn's disease. It did not help Shoshana, but the information was useful; lupus symptoms will almost always improve with such treatment. More reason, I thought, to look elsewhere for a cause.

Her father read about a new treatment for lupus, recently available, much talked about in the news.

"Can we try that?" he asked.

"I don't see why we would," I replied. "I do not think Shoshana has lupus. The drug is very expensive. There are clear guidelines for who should get this drug. The tests that confirm lupus must be positive; hers are negative. She does not fit the other guidelines. The drug is very new and very powerful; I don't know what it will do to her after years." And on and on.

"You've got to do something," her father countered. "She's wasting away. Her life will be destroyed."

Her father is a well-known doctor, powerful in his own field, a field that seldom treats patients with lupus. His arguments were logical and passionate, if not informed in this case. My protests did not dissuade him. After several more discussions like this, and because nothing I recommended seemed to help Shoshana, I acceded and wrote the prescription. To justify it I wrote the required ICD-9 code, 710.0, which I did not believe.

A few months later Shoshana was cured.

Or, to be accurate, she went into complete remission. Her pain stopped, the diarrhea ceased, her growth resumed.

That was several years ago. Today she is a confident and well young woman. As I write this she is living her junior college year in a foreign land. She continues treatment with the new drug. We will likely discontinue it one day, but not just now.

And—I am more humble with her father now.

I still do not think Shoshana has lupus. Even if she does, we violated the guidelines for use of the drug. I do not know why the medication worked so well. That is not important, because she is healthy again.

Diagnosis names and codes are just words and numbers, nothing more. I used the code number that would justify

Shoshana's prescription, not one I personally believed. The bureaucracy was happy and I was distraught, knowing that I had deceived, but pleased that I had helped my patient.

Years hence, when somebody reviews the use of this drug, that person will look only at the summary records that I submitted to the bureaucracy, not the details in my patient's office chart. No one will see the uncertain diagnosis and my misuse of the guidelines. The public record will say the treatment was successful for code 710.0. No one will check to see whether the code number matches the patient, and no one will see the uncertainty. The only questions asked will be whether the rules associated with 710.0 were followed, not whether the basic facts are, or are not, right.

17. Are Diagnosis Codes True?

Thinking about Shoshana, I began to think that many of my patients do not easily fit their assigned ICD codes. For them, standard treatment guidelines do not seem to apply.

I looked at my electronic records. The hand-held device on which I take patient notes holds information on about 500 patients at a time, so I looked at this convenient file to ask how many of my patients do not fit treatment guidelines.

On the day that I asked the question my device listed 518 patients. Two hundred eighteen of them, 42 percent, fell outside guideline rules. On a different day, for a different reason, I looked at a larger computer file of some 3000 patients. Twenty-five percent of those patients, and 44 percent of certain subgroups, fell outside guideline rules.

Why was this so?

Some had other diseases (like breast cancer) that made treatment by guidelines dangerous; some had rare diagnoses for which there are no guidelines; some, like most of the patients in these pages, had uncertain diagnoses; some for their own reasons refused guidelines-approved treatment; some had experienced intolerable side effects or allergy; others were pregnant, or took medicines that cannot be used together with those the guidelines advised; others simply refused.

Of course, I work at a specialty hospital in a medical center; we see many patients referred to us because their cases are complicated, so these patients may differ from those seen by other doctors. On the other hand, other doctors had seen these patients before I did, so they do exist in other practices. The proportion outside the guidelines may be higher in my practice, or not. I do not know.

Several weeks later I spoke at a large public meeting, an educational course for practicing doctors, about new developments in my field. As it happened, my speaking slot was early in the morning. My topic was what I have just been talking about: Patients who do not fit their codes, the first time I had chosen to speak publicly on this matter. Afterwards I sat in the lecture hall for the rest of the day because I was scheduled to give a second talk later on. To my surprise, every speaker (each from a different specialty) who followed me, citing me, *ad lib*bed comments about their own non-codable patients, or about those patients for whom guidelines did not apply. So, whatever the number, large or small, *all* doctors see these patients.

The real world is not as easily coded as the administrative committees that create these codes would have us believe. Our twenty-first century guidelines are irrelevant to many patients. Perhaps illnesses have lives of their own; perhaps they eschew the 141,742 separate names ICD-10 tries to give them; perhaps these illnesses have no sympathy with our bureaucratic rules.

* * * * *

The patient files I spoke of above, one with 518 patients, the other with 3,000, came from my past practice. Perhaps my practice has changed since then? Here are some examples from the past few weeks.

Last year Ellie, under someone else's care, almost died during a pregnancy complicated by an illness that I treat. Although she knew the problem would likely recur, she chose to become pregnant again. With her consent I prescribed an experimental treatment (not as part of a treatment trial, because there were no trials that would accept her) that I had reason to believe would help, but that her insurance would not support. She paid for the medication out of pocket. The pregnancy was filled with every anxiety her physicians could know. But, to her observation, the pregnancy was untroubled. She delivered a healthy child at full term. Two years on, I have just learned, a bit to my and her obstetrician's dismay, she wants to try for another child.

Dale and Anna, the young women I described in chapter 4, continue to come for follow-up care. They both have symptoms that fit many diagnoses simultaneously, what I call overlap disease, for which there are no treatment guidelines. There are guidelines for each of their individual diseases, but you cannot apply them together, since they contradict one another.

Having searched the Internet, Jennie ("I fit all the criteria!") asks me to prescribe a treatment that I consider dangerous and inappropriate, so I refuse. She goes to another doctor, tells him that I agreed (that is, lies to him about what I said) and gives him a credible reason why she left my care. He does not call me to verify; instead, he prescribes the treatment she requests. She then returns to me to handle the treatment's complications, so long, she says, as I promise to continue to prescribe it. (I did not prescribe the medication, because of the dangers she now could see, but she came back to my care and agreed to follow my advice.)

Stacy has severe symptoms. Her laboratory tests are equivocal. The guideline for treating what I think she has requires her to have positive tests. I prescribe the preferred, but expensive, treatment anyway, hoping her insurer will pay.

Doreen sought advice because a laboratory test suggested lupus. She has no symptoms now. The abnormal test had been found on a screening panel that had no reason to have been done. Chances are that she will never fall ill. The treatment I might offer (if there were reason to treat) will have severe side effects. To me this discussion is easy, because I cannot predict she will ever be ill, nor can I prevent illness from occurring, if that is to be her fate. I will, I tell her, treat symptoms if and when they occur. I suggest that the best option is to wait. She rejects that advice. She leaves my practice to find another doctor who will treat her as she asks.

Lou, a man in his forties, is intellectually challenged and possibly mentally ill. His mother, now aged and disabled herself, comes with him to my office because he cannot recall conversations or follow instructions on his own. I cannot prescribe anything that has complicated instructions or that requires a patient to report unusual effects.

Manjulika, pregnant and nearly crippled with rheumatoid arthritis, lives a secret, subsistence life. She is an undocumented immigrant with no health insurance. The medical decisions should be easy, but she needs to stay hidden from immigration authorities, so I keep a private medical chart, not in the hospital records, and I do not submit paperwork that might put her at risk for deportation. The best medication for her is very expensive. With assistance from our Social Services department I identify a no-questions-asked compassionate-care program that will supply the medications she needs. I work with an obstetrician who agrees to help with her care.

Saeeda, a young foreign physician who does have a legal work visa, has just developed rheumatoid arthritis. She had come to this country to begin a medical internship, which will begin in a few months, and which will provide health insurance. She had come early to learn to be more comfortable with Western ways and to adjust to American English. Meanwhile she volunteers in a research laboratory nearby, with no insurance. She needs treatment now. Will she be able to hold out until her job begins?[14]

These people are not rare. I saw them all in just the past few weeks. None of them can be treated by guidelines, because treatment is: Unconventional (Ellie); without guidelines (Dale and Anna); inappropriate (Jennie and Doreen); refused because of criteria that are too rigid (Stacy); impossible because of mental/intellectual concerns (Lou); or restricted by socioeconomic rules (Manjulika and Saeeda).

Yes, guidelines are for the most part evidence-based. Yes, the point of guidelines is to protect patients.

No, diagnoses do not follow guideline rules. Individual patients present problems that guidelines cannot predict.

---

[14] A few weeks later Manjulika lost the pregnancy and then disappeared again into the illegal immigrant underground. The same compassionate-care program provided medication for Saeeda as it had for Manjulika.

Yes, I know criteria and guidelines. I will follow them if I can. It is just that forty-two percent of my patients do not fit those rules.

Part V. To Define a Diagnosis

18. A Mouse Falls Ill

To truly understand a disease, we use mice.

Except for the "ick" factor, mice are wonderful beasts. They are available to researchers by the thousands, in all sorts of colors and sizes. They are cheap and easy to raise. They have big litters, so it is easy to compare mouse siblings treated in different ways.

You can change a mouse's genes, even give it human genes. You can breed mice to have specific illnesses and you can use mice to test treatments. You can change a mouse's diet and change its germs to see what will happen to them and, by analogy, to humans who are ill.

In many ways, mice are perfect models of human disease. This is not a secret. Almost everything we think about an illness—its origins, its mechanisms, its cures—can be studied in a mouse.

But there are a few differences between mice and men.

- Mice do not take three trains to see their doctors. In fact, doctors make house calls to them.

- A mouse does not have a problem being a single mom.

- Mice are not homeless.

- They do not try herbal remedies that their cousins recommend.

- They do not (usually) use alcohol or cocaine.

- A mouse bred to have a specific disease will not also have asthma, or pancreatitis, or stroke, or diabetes, or any other—we call it co-morbid—illness as well.

- Mice do not have insurers who refuse to pay for an out-of-network doctor. In fact, mice are never uninsured.

- Mice are not illegal immigrants.

- Mice do not refuse to take a drug because it causes weight gain.

- Most mice who are ill will not have just returned from a three-week safari trip in Kenya or a beach vacation in Thailand.

- Most mice studied have not been ill for the mouse equivalent of forty years, nor have they been treated with different and now obsolete treatments throughout that time.

- Mice do not eat Chinese food on Tuesday, Mexican on Saturday, and Big Macs in-between.

- Mice do not have college roommates who are impossible.

- Mice do not drop out of school to find themselves, or return after a year abroad.

- Mice do not take birth control pills.

- Mice are not on food stamps. In fact, they seldom go hungry.

Of course, I concede that some mice are subject to domestic violence. On the other hand, animal care regulations set rules about the maximum number of mice allowed to live in one room, about how big their living spaces must be, about the temperatures of their living spaces, and about how they should be fed.

I concede their physicians do not have the mice's best interests at heart. Their doctors seldom treat a mouse's other illnesses (if such ever occur), not even an antihistamine for allergies or an acetaminophen tablet for fever; they never administer acupuncture or mixtures of herbs. If a mouse is anxious, it does not see a therapist. Mice rarely get routine immunizations, certainly not for the mouse version of annual flu. Doctors never put mice in intensive care units, bring them back from near death, and treat them if they fall ill again. In fact, the mouse's doctor will probably kill his sick patient instead.

So far as we know, a mouse does not think about its symptoms or talk about them with family members for months before it decides to seek care. A mouse does not refuse a prescription based on personal belief or religion or a neighbor's anecdotes of a terrible experience with the same drug. Insurers do not refuse to pay for the treatment that a mouse's doctor deems best. Whether a drug affects fertility, causes fetal malformations, or causes acne or mood changes or weight gain is of no concern to a mouse at all. And never, ever, does a mouse have to decide who is correct among doctors who disagree. A medical history and a physical examination for a mouse are straightforward. In fact, a mouse never gives a confusing history or lies about unusual sexual habits, a prior abortion, or drug use that it does not choose to reveal.

For humans, different doctors see and hear different things in the same patient. Some patients and doctors talk easily to one another; others do not. Not so for mice. A mouse may distrust its doctor, may run to the corner of its cage, and may even bite, but it cannot refuse to do what the doctor prescribes.

Mice cannot model those non-medical things that affect ill humans. We think that the biology of disease is the most important thing. Mice are good models for that. We ignore the externalities that affect an illness. Mice are terrible models for that.

The external things that affect a human, but not a mouse, are many. How much the patient can afford; what are the patient's responsibilities (to home, family, culture, and job); how long does it take to get to appointments; what are the conveniences, attitudes, and dangers of a patient's neighborhood; what will the insurer allow; what will the patient's religion or culture allow; in what country was the patient born; what are the diet preferences and diet rules; whether the patient has another illness or injury or genetic abnormality that will affect the plan; whether she is pregnant; if she is exposed to environmental and workplace risks, like sunlight, or mold, or pollen, or pollution— all these things affect how a patient responds to illness. They do not affect the illness of a mouse.

19. Process and Cause

Naming, counting, accepting the scales of Time—these are the structural elements of uncertainty. We use these elements to study the process of a disease, not its cause.

What is process? What is cause?

We say that a cholesterol deposit in a coronary artery is the cause of a heart attack, that a virus is the cause of flu, that smoking is the cause of lung cancer. A cause: The thing at the very beginning that sets everything in motion, the thing without which nothing will happen. Without which, nothing. *Sine qua, non.*

This is logical: If you remove the cause, you can prevent a disease. If the disease is underway, by attacking the cause you may be able to effect its cure. You can target your therapy to that single aim. No cause, no disease. Right?

Maybe not. Knowing when a disease begins is not always certain. Why or how did the cholesterol get in the artery? Where did the virus come from, and how did it come to you?

Was is in your body for a long while, dormant, and did something happen that released it from its lair?

A while ago I saw a nice metaphor to explain cause (I do not remember where). When you flip a light switch, what causes the light to go on? Is it the flipping of the switch or something more?

Consider this: In geological time, mountains rise. The earth turns. The earth has a tilt as it circles the sun, so we have night and day and seasons, times of warmth and times of cold. Because the earth turns and because the temperature changes the atmosphere moves. Moisture is in the air, and snow falls on the mountains. The snow melts and becomes water, which gives us rivers, which, falling down mountains, power mills. Through generators the mills make electricity, which is "tamed" by high voltage transformers, carried over wires to substations, "tamed" further by low voltage transformers, carried by other wires into your building, and distributed to a circuit that contains a light bulb and a switch. You flip the switch. The light bulb shines. The mountains, the earth turning, the earth's tilt, the rivers.... You get the point. They are all "causes" that make the light bulb go on.

The story continues. Why, at the beginning, does snow fall? At the end, who invented the light bulb? Who made the bulb you put in your lamp? For that matter, who made the lamp and the socket? Who sold it? Who bought it? Who inserted it? Who installed the wires?

Then you depend on your eyes to see darkness change to light. Your eyes send that message to the back of the brain, which tells your conscious mind: The light shines.

So what is the "cause" of the light turning on? The switch? The mountain? The sun? The bulb maker? The lamp seller? Your brain? Or everything in between?

What the "cause" is cannot fully be known. It is the process that we understand—the transition between snow and river, the change of energy state that makes the filament glow—not the cause. Each step, from the snow on the mountain to the switch to the bulb in the lamp, is one small part of a process. Target and block any single one of those parts, jam the waterwheel, burn the transformer, cut the wire, remove the bulb, remove any one of those things: No light will shine. Process is not cause. It is more important, or at least more understandable, than cause.

So with the processes of disease. The bulb shines or does not or burns weakly: Metaphors for a cure, a death, or something in-between. Block a process and the illness stops. Healing begins.

Perhaps someday we will know the "cause" of chronic illnesses, but today we treat patients by correcting or mitigating abnormal processes, like inflammation or abnormal blood clotting. The cause remains. If the waterwheel breaks, a nuclear reactor may provide electricity. If the body finds a way to bypass the treatment (the factor that mitigates the process) the symptoms may return. Or other problems may occur. The nuclear reactor may contaminate the land. Bypass a damaged wire, a short circuit may cause a fire. Block one disease process, a different problem may take its place. Yet it is easier to know—and to intervene in—process than it is to eradicate a cause.

20. Qualitative, Quantitative

In chapter 6 I cited the case of the lady in the *New England Journal of Medicine* CPC, who had a strange rash. Did I mention that the lady was black? Did I mention that, in the words of the CPC, "For religious reasons, she was reluctant to take medications and was distrustful of the medical system"?

These parts of a patient's story are almost always ignored in the medical charts, clinical research, diagnostic codes, guidelines, and algorithms on which our practices are based, but they are important. What is also important, these ignored aspects can be analyzed, qualitatively and quantitatively.

Qualitative, quantitative. Though these words sound like jargon, they mean only simple logic and organized thought. To understand something, define it. Define, characterize, describe: That is *qualitative* thinking. After defining that thing, measure and weigh it: That is *quantitative* thinking. For diagnosis and treatment, the point is to consider the patient's symptoms and findings both ways.

The qualitative parts of this patient's story are that she distrusts the medical system, is religious, and, in this case, is black in a mostly white world. The quantitative part is to assign a weight to each qualitative part.

So let us assign weights to qualities. Distrust, for discussion purposes, give it an arbitrary weight of ten; religious beliefs, assign a weight of two; race conflicts, a weight of five, according to how much effect you believe each quality will have on the final medical decision.

I made up these numbers, of course, but I need not have done. Social sciences instruct us how to assign such weights to social factors, make them quantitative, that is. The numbers I made up are for purposes of illustration about how such a calculation might be done. You can add the points for each quality to calculate their effect on the patient's prognosis.

Assigning weights to qualities in order to solve problems quantitatively is something that scientists do. When you quantify something you can build complex mathematical equations of relationships, and then use those equations to predict outcomes. This is done every day, as when molecular geneticists predict the effects of several simultaneously active genes on a patient's health. Today's computers handle these complex calculations quite well. In genetics, molecular biology, and all the health sciences, computer models that calculate strengths of relationships are commonplace.[x] One can look at hundreds of processes at once, quantitatively, simultaneously or sequentially, see how much effect each has at each step, and predict the end result that is caused by a change in any, or many, of the parts.

Researchers in the basic sciences are taught always to think quantitatively. Clinicians think about patients mostly qualitatively, but they also think quantitatively, often unconsciously. When they predict the course of an illness they do so by instinct. This patient has a fever and rash: A qualitative thought. The fever is very important, the rash less so: A quantitative thought. To estimate from today's kidney function test the date a patient will have to start dialysis or receive a kidney transplant is quantitative. To predict a bad outcome when you see a large tumor mass in a brain MRI is qualitative.

Clinicians tend to focus, qualitatively and quantitatively, on a disease's biology, blood tests, biopsies, and X-rays. They often ignore the quantifiable aspects of a patient's social, historical, environmental, and belief structures. As with genes and molecules, one can assign numbers to social and personal things—lack of insurance, a sexual relationship, or travel time to an appointment. One can say that such a factor has no influence (score it zero), a little, a moderate amount, or a lot (score one, two, or three). One can give a score for fundamentalist belief, for being caregiver to a parent with Alzheimer's, and many other things, so as to calculate the effect of that item on a person's health. These non-biological influences affect a patient's choice to seek care, to take medications, and to recover as surely as does the effect of gene A on gene B. They affect the likelihood a patient will heal. I can cite many more things that influence health, and I can make reasonable guesses about how much they should weigh. In fact, I have made such guesses with my patients.

Here are items I would weigh: The patient's heritage, marital status, relationships, and living and work situations. I would assign weights to her medical history, recent and remote, and to whether she is pregnant or not our hopes or fears to be. I would consider the effect of Time: The longer a problem has been present, the more damage will have accrued.

With regard to biology of disease, some measures are easily counted—temperature, pulse rate, abnormal blood tests, counts of swollen joints. Others are not. How does one measure severity of a headache or of fatigue, of itching or pain? In reality, it is not hard. As with the social issues, simple English suffices. None, mild, moderate, severe. Zero, one, two, three.

To measure severity of illness quantitatively, create a plausible list and sum the numbers. A patient with a low score is less ill, one with a high score more so. The score will suggest a prognosis: Low score, likely recovery; high score, likely not. The score will measure how effective treatment is. If the score goes down, the treatment worked or remission occurred. If the score goes up, the treatment failed.

21. Muddle

Doctors do use the kinds of criteria, indices, and algorithms discussed in chapter 15, at least for the biological aspects of disease. These indices seldom include the personal variables I bring up here.

One disease activity index for lupus that most American doctors use is called the SLEDAI.[15] SLEDAI measures biology: Symptoms and laboratory tests. In SLEDAI, a seizure gets eight points, arthritis four, protein in the urine four, and fever one point. (These are just examples; there are many more ways for a patient to acquire points.) The sum of all the points scored on a given day gives the SLEDAI score for that day. The higher the sum, the worse the patient is.

I decided that a fairer summary should also include social, historical, and environmental elements, so I invented my own index. I called it "Muddle," for MDLLE (my initials, MDL,

---

[15] Pronounced "slee-dye", for Systemic Lupus Erythematosus Disease Activity Index. The British, of course, have their own index, called BILAG, for British Isles Lupus Activity Group.

plus L̲upus E̲xercise). The "Muddle" index is fantasy, for my personal amusement, or perhaps for my personal edification. I did not tell anybody about "Muddle" nor ask others to use it, but the thought did cross my mind. Like SLEDAI, "Muddle" distinguishes between, and gives separate weights to, symptoms (what a patient feels, like pain or nausea) and signs (physical abnormalities, like fever or a swollen joint). Unlike SLEDAI, "Muddle" assigns a weight to both biologic and non-biologic factors like those mentioned in Chapter 20.

To test "Muddle," I invented two different patients, imaginary, but I see patients like these every day. I named one R.D., for *Rich District* and the other I.C., for *Inner City*. I scored their visits side-by-side, both by SLEDAI and by "Muddle".

On the SLEDAI score R.D. and I.C. look very much alike.[xi]

Unlike SLEDAI, "Muddle," gives additional points for bad genes (a modern addition that is impractical to measure in SLEDAI). To simplify things, I decided to give R.D. and I.C. the same bad genes, so, on the basis of assigned points, they still look alike.

I made R.D. older. Since age worsens prognosis, R.D. looks a bit worse. I.C.'s heritage is African, a factor that makes her prognosis worse, so she gets these points. She has been ill longer, more points. R.D. has easy access to medical care. I.C. does not, so I.C. gets more points. I.C. has a cousin and an aunt with lupus (the disease tends to run in families), R.D. does not, so again the score is against I.C. Patient R.D. has good health habits, goes to a gym, watches her diet. I.C. has no access to gyms, eats fast foods, and is overweight. I.C. smokes and once or twice tried cocaine. R.D. has done neither. The numbers continue to favor R.D.

Fairly or not, doctors call some patients "non-compliant", meaning they do not follow the doctor's orders. Compliance is a matter of mutual trust, of willingness to accept unpleasant side effects, and of the ability to buy medications. It is hard to find this information in a medical chart, but sometimes you know. In this case R.D. trusts the medical profession and can easily get her medications, so she gets no points. I.C. goes to a clinic rather than to a private doctor's office, where she sees a different resident (trainee) doctor each time. She thinks many of them are fools. I.C. has heard a lot about the Tuskegee syphilis experiments,[xii] and everybody she knows is talking about Henrietta Lacks,[xiii] so she gets more points for distrust. She does not take medications that make her feel ill; sometimes she does not have enough money to fill her prescriptions; and sometimes her local pharmacy does not carry the drug. She is, we say, "non-compliant" (more points).

I did the formal calculations for both patients by SLEDAI and by "Muddle". If SLEDAI were your measure, these women are much alike: They have similar symptoms and similar blood tests. If "Muddle" is the measure, by heritage, habit, family, trust, access to medication and many other things, I.C. scores many more points than does R.D.

So who has a better prognosis? If both R.D. and I.C. participate in the same clinical trial of a new drug, which woman is more likely to do well?

SLEDAI counts only the biology of a disease. "Muddle," to my way of thinking, is more true. It is not necessary to understand *how* the extra "Muddle" points affect outcome, the qualitative part. For the time being, knowing *how much* effect, the quantitative part, they have will suffice. Make the qualitative information quantitative and you will understand more.

The concept behind "Muddle" is not new. Doctors have always known that social and personal factors are important in medical care. It is commonplace in doctors' conversations to hear, "I gave her a prescription but she didn't take it," or, "She says she ran out of her medicines two months ago! Again!"

I see patients in my private office and in our outpatient Medicaid clinic. Each week at the clinic conference I listen with head-shaking dismay as I hear about the difficulty disadvantaged patients have in obtaining the same care that those with better fortune can access easily—and in even more dismay when I hear some doctors yell at these patients for not overcoming obstacles they themselves have never had to face. When we ask these patients to participate in research projects, we score them all by the SLEDAI index, and think there is little difference between those we see in the clinic and those we see in our private practices. Would we think the same if we had scored them by "Muddle"?

Seeing non-compliance, doctors intuitively think, "This patient will not do well," but they rarely record such information in a patient's medical chart, and it is rare for such information to appear in reports of clinical trials. Those who devise best-practice guidelines pay the "Muddle" Index items little heed.

In some future day, I believe, doctors will be obliged to weigh the non-biologic factors in their assessments of severity and prognosis. Someday they may even include these factors when they interpret their treatment trials. The social and economic factors of illness affect outcome at least as much as does a misbehaving gene. To measure these factors is not beyond our ken. We can name, count, and weigh the factors. In the clinic as well as in the research laboratory, we can think quantitatively and qualitatively. We can describe and weigh what we do not know. Thus we create a roadmap by which we can use—not hide from—uncertainty, in our quest to reach our goal.

22. The Music in the Words

Many years ago, in college, I read (or tried to read) *The Waste Land*, T. S. Eliot's epic post-World War I poem about sorrow and loss. Eliot reveled in obscure references. Throughout his poem he scattered quotes in foreign languages, sometimes in scripts other than Roman. The poem's beginning is almost completely uninterpretable to a modern reader. Its prologue is a quotation from Gaius Petronius' *The Satyricon*, a satire written in Latin in the first century C.E. that describes an episode in which Sybil, a prophetess of Apollo, hanging in a cage, contests her capture. Eliot quotes her speech in the original Latin and switches to Greek, in Greek orthography, when her Greek captors talk. [xiv] Except to the professors who assigned the poem to my college class and to the academics who have written hundreds if not thousands of papers about the poem, and to a few others who understand both Latin and Greek and *The Satyricon* (I suppose such people do exist), the beginning of *The Waste Land* may be the very definition of opacity.

The last stanza of Eliot's poem begins in Italian (not just any Italian, but a quote from Dante). Not much better. The next line is a mysterious reference in English, "O Swallow, Swallow", which appears to come from Tennyson's *The Princess* (thank you, Google and Wikipedia), and the next line is an equally obscure line in French, *Le prince d'Aquitaine à la tour abolie*, (the Prince of Aquitaine at the ruined tower). This is the Prince to whom I pay homage in the title of this book. The remaining lines of Eliot's poem, presented in archaic English and Sanskrit, are equally obscure.

At least I could read most of the middle parts of *The Waste Land*. Obscurity aside, the poem is powerful. Who does not know its famous first line:

April is the cruellest month?[xv]

Obscure, yes, but something solid and clear as well.

In college I had no idea what *The Waste Land*'s last few stanzas meant, or what the references were to, or why Eliot insisted on writing in multiple languages. The only thing that made any sense to me at all was the line in French, "*Le prince d'Aquitaine à la tour abolie*," which I knew from other reading to be a line of a poem written by the mid-19th century romantic poet, Gérard de Nerval.

Knowing the source for that line did not help me understand what the Prince of Aquitaine meant to either Eliot or de

Nerval, particularly because de Nerval's poem itself had its own mysteries. Though he wrote in French, he gave his poem a title, *El Desdichado*, using an outdated Spanish term that means the downtrodden one, or the scorned one.

Who was *El Desdichado*? A specific person? Why was the title in Spanish rather than in French? I had no idea and de Nerval does not say. And who was the Prince of Aquitaine? What tower was he at? Why had the tower collapsed? Or perhaps the English cognate of *abolie*, abolished, would be a more to-the-point translation. Passive verb structure. Why was the tower abolished? By whom? The de Nerval poem does not answer these questions. It brings up the thought and leaves it hanging in the air.

This is how de Nerval's poem, *El Desdichado*, begins:

Je suis le ténébreux, - le veuf, - l'inconsolé,
Le prince d'Aquitaine à la tour abolie[xvi]

In translation:

I am the one of the black mood, the widower, the unconsoled one
The Prince of Aquitaine at the ruined tower

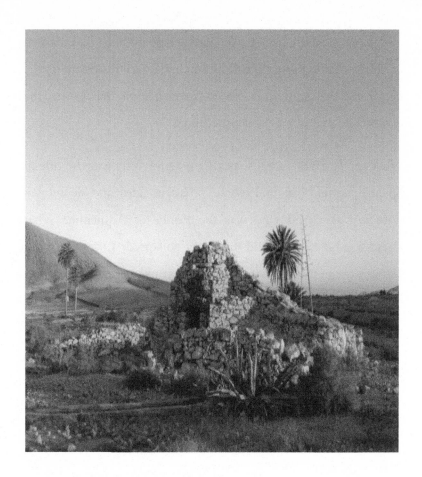

A Ruined Tower (photo Miriam Lockshin)

After that the poem drops all further mention of the Prince and goes on to describe the writer's despondency and desolation.

I have read and re-read Eliot and I have read and re-read de Nerval. I still have no idea who the Prince was or why the tower was torn down. Nor, for that matter, did I have any idea why Eliot found it important to quote de Nerval's line, or, why he chose to do so at the poem's end?

For no reason that I could understand, despite its complete obscurity, the line about the Prince stayed with me. Periodically I would hear the refrain in my head, uttered in sonorous baritone voice, almost a song, in the tonal changes of French cadence. I still hear it today. The line seems to me a deep statement of sadness and of what cannot be known.

As I was thinking about the meanings of patient histories, of what we doctors do and do not understand, the words "*Le prince d'Aquitaine à la tour abolie*" returned to me, and with them the sounds and the puzzle from my college days. So I Googled the words, "Prince of Aquitaine."

Well, yes, I did find a fair amount of history about the Prince of Aquitaine (or the Princes—there were several famous ones, it seems—as well as a few Princesses). But I found nothing about a ruined tower except references to de Nerval's and Eliot's poems. I did find that many others continue to debate the meaning of those lines.

Perhaps the best answer—at least the one to which I felt closest—was written by Richard Sieburth, a professor and translator, in an introduction to his translation of de Nerval.[xvii] As a student, he, like me, had been struck by that line. He writes that he often declaimed it out loud, as I had done silently, not knowing what its meaning might be. Eventually he concluded that the meaning is in the music, not the sense, of the line. Declaimed in French, *Le prince d'Aquitaine à la tour abolie* is almost a song.

The line transmits emotion, not information. It is not important who the Prince was, which tower fell or was torn down, or why de Nerval chose a Spanish title, for a poem in French, that speaks of sadness and loss.

It is so obvious now. How could I not have known?

23. A Real Life Tale

Medical histories are a bit like the line from de Nerval that Eliot cites. Patient and doctor may agree on what is said, but it is the music as much as the words that convey meaning. What the patient intends and what the doctor hears, what the doctor means and what the patient understands, are never the same. The meaning lies in how the patient speaks as much as in what she says. It is the job of the doctor to hear the music within.

Doctors have two duties: To diagnose and to prescribe. From Hippocrates to Galen, from Ibn Sina to Maimonides, and up to this very day, symptoms and diagnosis, prescription and cure, that has been the rule.

Except for two problems. What is the gold standard for a medical history? And do patients do what they are told?

A history of an illness is not a fixed thing. The speaker will think one fact important, another irrelevant; the doctor may think otherwise. A probing question here, a chance comment by a spouse, a glance, a shift in posture, a phrase that can be interpreted in two ways. Something forgotten. Something else recalled. Who is hurried, who is not. An unexpected word, a physical examination finding that triggers a memory from long ago. Mutual trust or suspicion. Many things alter the discourse.

I learned this rather rudely as, planning retirement, I transferred my patients to my younger (female) colleague. I learned that, for many of my patients, I was a father figure, while my colleague was their friend.

To which one of us, me or my colleague, would Claudia (chapter 8) cry about her breakup with a boyfriend, or talk about that boyfriend at all? Which of us could read in a change of make-up or dress a change in the direction of a patient's life? To which of us would a young patient confess that she had stopped taking medications? On the other hand, which of us could recognize a rash normally seen only in Brazil, or would associate darkened ear lobes with a metabolic disease? Different physicians see different things. No single one of us can see it all.

As a medical resident I became the physician of a patient whose previous physician had thought her "very fidgety" (wrote those exact words in his sign-off chart note). But she was not fidgety—she had Huntington's chorea, an hereditary brain disease that causes unintended movement, the connection invisible to one doctor, obvious to the next. We all can be blind to such clues. This is not a flaw specific to doctors; rather, it is a human flaw. We all can have tunnel vision. We all, at some time or at all times, see only what we expect to see. Or we draw different lessons from what we do see.

A new patient came in today. Taking his history, I thought the fact of a rare disease in his mother and grandmother was an important clue. A colleague, himself well-known and highly competent, knows that history and thinks it irrelevant. I do not know which of us is right.

A few days ago I listened to the detailed medical history of a new patient. She had not brought with her, and I had no access to, her prior medical records. Startled at what her other doctors seemed to have missed, at the end of the consultation I suggested what seemed to me an obvious diagnosis and possible cure. The patient then said, offhandedly, "Oh, I forgot to tell you. I tried all that five years ago." Had she not belatedly recalled her past, the note I was about to write would have startled other doctors by what I seemed to have missed.

If you believe medical textbooks, answers are always simple. A history, an examination, and a few tests lead to a diagnosis. A diagnosis leads to a prescription; a prescription leads to a result. Textbooks rarely acknowledge that any medical history reflects the chosen emphases of both the speaker and the recorder, that different examiners note different things, that the lines drawn between diagnoses are not always clear, that symptoms and illnesses change over time, and that outcomes can be judged differently by different observers, including the patient herself.

This is why my friend and colleague called: His distant medical school had recruited a physician, a professor at another medical school near to us, to be chairman of one of his school's departments. The recruited doctor's wife had stayed in New York for the nonce, pending their child's graduation from high school. She had begun to have episodes of great fatigue that other doctors had been unable to explain. My colleague was calling on behalf of his new recruit to ask if I would help sort this out.

A bit puzzled, I said yes, but unenthusiastically. The complaint had seemed vague. Clearly her episodes of fatigue had occurred simultaneously with a major life change, the move to a distant place. I did not personally know the family, and I had no reason to think one thing or another, but it is obvious that such changes can allow emotions to dominate a physical complaint.

Though I assumed that my colleague did not choose my name at random, if there was a specific reason for the consulting doctor to be me, or any rheumatologist, he did not say. Perhaps he was not at liberty to elaborate, or perhaps there was some other private concern. Oh, well. Acceding to this kind of request is what friends and colleagues do.

Another reason for my lack of enthusiasm was that it is not easy to treat the families of doctors. Some of their relatives want to be seen at the first hint of something wrong, presenting barely recognizable symptoms, and they focus compulsively on what are (to me) minor issues, below my threshold to diagnose or treat. Others come with advanced disease that could or should have been prevented or controlled, but whose unmistakable warning signs had been ignored, for whatever reason, by the physician-relative (but sometimes by the patient) for immeasurable lengths of now lost time.

This is the reason the lady gave for her visit: She was having episodes of weakness, characterized by profound fatigue and possibly breathlessness. Sometimes her joints hurt, a complaint that had been true for years. A few months earlier she had a transient rash. More recently she had an episode of chest pain that lasted several days. She saw a cardiologist who thought the cause was not in his field. She saw a lung specialist who said it was not in his. However, he gave her medications for asthma, just in case. The patient said the asthma medicines may have helped. Then she said, offhandedly, almost in a whisper, with a hint of embarrassment, that sometimes she felt unsteady. "I walk like a drunk," she said.

As she said this she looked down to her right and away, then changed the subject. The unsteadiness was not why she came. She appeared not to want to discuss it further.

I found her manner curious and so I decided to probe. It seems what she called weakness was unsteadiness of gait. Feeling about to fall, she thought her muscles were giving way. I do not know why that admission embarrassed her—clearly there were thoughts she did not wish to share—but once the topic was broached she became expansive. She spoke of other rashes (she had photographs on her cell phone to show), of changes in her sweating patterns, and of other strange symptoms she would have preferred to ignore.

Those symptoms were not incidental. Like an intoxicated driver in a roadside police test, she failed every test of physical coordination that I know how to do. Even before I ordered an MRI, I suspected that she had a serious brain disease. The asthma medicines she had begun to take contain a substantial amount of corticosteroid, which can improve some types of brain inflammation, so her response perhaps was no surprise.

Why do I tell this tale? In part to say that if you take a patient's complaint only at face value—"I have episodes of weakness"— if you do not see the accompanying emotion, if you do not then probe and reinterpret, you may miss essential facts.

This may be a story of failed translation. Perhaps she did not have the words to describe what she felt, or, being used to doctors but not trained in our vocabulary herself, she used words she thought were right but that confused me and others. Whatever the reason, her words misled. I had to translate her speech, tease from "weakness" its constituent parts ("instability") and then put it into my own, usable and actionable, vocabulary ("ataxia").

Something about the instability seemed to embarrass her, and so she had tried to keep that symptom to herself. I met her just a few days ago and do not yet know what that something might be. Perhaps as I get to know her better, she will explain.[16]

Whatever the tests, now pending, will disclose, for now the quick, averted look, the unexpected change of topic, and the moment of hesitant speech tells me more about her symptoms than do her words. I would have been superficial, callous, or unthinking had I dismissed or avoided confronting that which she seemed to wish to avoid. That I understand.

This is what I do not understand. I was the third doctor the patient saw. Did those other doctors consider only diagnoses that their specialties know? Could they not think of possibilities beyond?

---

[16] I did not have to intuit an answer. Later she told me that the way I asked my question (so much for the doctor being a neutral party to this conversation) told her I was not talking about a likely transient illness, which she thought it was, but about something potentially serious and possibly progressive. She suddenly understood that what I was asking about involved her brain and that her future and her life were under threat. The looking away had not been embarrassment, but terror. It seems I heard the music but my interpretation had been off-key. The tests we then did showed a transient type of brain inflammation that we could and did successfully treat.

I can see only two answers to those questions. The first is that the other doctors, for lack of time, confidence, or imagination, could not exit their comfort zones. The second is that, missing the askew glance, ignoring the change in tone, they failed to see the music hidden in her words.

Part VI. To Solve the Problem

24. Breaching Barriers

For doctor and patient to understand, negotiate about, and work with uncertainty, they must first establish a common language. Communication is not automatic. Try as I may to overcome missed communication with "Muddle," I still meet boundaries of culture, education, and language that overwhelm understanding. It is difficult to hear music when its style crosses vast personal and cultural terrains. Yet even though the differences are enormous, it is possible for very different people to talk.

If you saw only the notes in her medical chart, you might think that Chantal is not a nice person. If the notes are your only evidence, you would probably be right.

She did not trust doctors, whose mistakes, she said, had killed her mother. Chantal often ended her clinic visits in argument. Doctors wanted to experiment on her, she said. They ordered her to do things that she could not in conscience do. Doctors yelled at her, she said, and she yelled back.

The disputes were dramatic and public. Once, in hospital for a medical crisis, an unknown someone in a white coat had lectured her (again) for her intransigence. That evening, after the lights dimmed, Chantal took a Magic Marker, scrawled obscenities on the hospital room's walls, and disappeared into the night. "Left against medical advice," the chart note said, not omitting a lurid description of the very visible facts. Chantal trusted only one doctor, one who was still in training, who addressed her as Mrs. and not by her first name, and who did not yell back.

Chantal found herself pregnant at a particularly bad time—her kidneys and heart were quite weak; her disease raged through her body uncontrolled. The obstetricians advised her to end the pregnancy. The cardiologists were more direct and dictatorial: They ordered her to undergo abortion, threatening not to treat her, to fire her from their clinic, if she refused. The doctor Chantal trusted offered to support her, whatever she chose to do.

When the cardiologist ordered Chantal to terminate the pregnancy, a very loud shouting match erupted in the middle of the clinic. Peacemakers and hospital ethicists rushed to intervene. Calm restored, they called for a meeting of all of us (I was her doctor's supervisor) to discuss the concerns.

We doctors—cardiologists, obstetricians, rheumatologists alike—concurred in this: The pregnancy would be difficult. Indeed, we all agreed, Chantal might not survive. If she did, very likely she would not live to see her child grown.

Chantal's answer was this: "Whether I live or die is not the point. I have been sick for years. I will die one day. What I do is important to me, not to you. Whether I have the child or not, I will still be ill. If I don't have this child, my life will mean nothing. This child will say that my life mattered. It is my decision, not yours. Your job is to help me succeed."

Brava!

Whether what followed was good or bad depends upon your point of view. A few months later Chantal, nearing the end of the pregnancy, was admitted to our medical intensive care unit (ICU) with a failing heart. A short while later, still in the ICU, she delivered a healthy boy. She remained in the ICU for a few more weeks, but eventually went home to care for her newborn son.

In the quiet moments of those long hospital days and of the later clinic visits that followed, Chantal shared with her doctor and me, and with a social worker to whom she had become close, the better moments of her life. She showed us videos of songs that she wrote and sang with her friends. She shared with us the draft of a book she was writing, about living a full life despite the threat of imminent death.

When she came to our clinic in the months that followed we saw her beautiful, peaceful smile, as, waiting to be called to the examination room, she sat on the floor and played with her son.

Chantal did die few years later. By that time it had been a very long time since we had seen her anger. Instead, on her clinic days, she greeted us with hugs. We hugged her, and her son, in return.

If you saw only the notes in her medical chart, you might think Chantal was not a nice person. You would be wrong. She was a very nice person. That day in the clinic when she and the cardiologists argued, Chantal taught, to every doctor and nurse who was there, what dignity means.

For teaching us these lessons, Chantal became one of the heroes we honored in the ceremony described in Chapter 11.

25. To Understand One Another

In 2009 Alida Brill and I wrote a book together, called *Dancing at the River's Edge*.[xviii] Alida has been my patient and friend for many years. Trained as an academic social critic, she has the tools and the vocabulary to describe how patients and doctors talk to one another. The book is structured as a dialogue between us two, contrapuntal chapters about specific episodes in her life, and about what she or I felt, saw, and heard at that particular time.

Mostly we agreed on what we each had thought. Sometimes one of us was startlingly wrong. We did not see at the time how we misunderstood one another.

The details of the misunderstandings are not the point. The question is: If we, alert to, even focused on, doctor-patient dialogue, repeatedly mistook one another, how do patients and doctors who share little communicate at all? How do they talk across age, race, heritage, wealth, education, and even gaps in language that are potentially huge? How does a white, older, middle-class, establishment-educated doctor talk to a young, poor, black, distrustful Chantal (Chapter 24), and how does she explain to me what she feels? Even bypassing the racial and economic differences, given my age and my sex, I will never be a best friend to a teen-age girl. I do not think I will ever notice a changed hair style, a scarf, or matching fingernails, eye shadow, and shoes. A doctor in a rich hospital's clinic will never hear all that a poor person has on her mind.

Yet there are moments when barriers are overcome. Amirah (Chapter 5) looked directly into my eyes. Chantal reached out for a hug.

Dancing at the River's Edge is not a long book. It begins with the child Alida's story of how she first understood that she was always going to be a patient. She devised mental magical tricks to pretend she was well. She learned how to command control of her visits with a new doctor. To make the right impression, she used posturing and pretense and sometimes half-truths. She knew which words and actions would trigger a desired or a feared response. She knew how to structure the interview to be certain that the doctor would accede to her lead.

As a young doctor, I also learned to structure first interviews, to avoid comments that I judged frightening, to reassure, to decide what to reveal and what to hide. I used posturing and pretense and sometimes half-truths.

In private, Alida judges her doctors, sometimes humorously, sometimes with devastating brutality. She does not offer her negative opinions out loud. Using polite subterfuge and deception, Alida communicates her wishes to her doctor. Using blunt, angry, and impolite words, Chantal did the same. For my part, like most doctors (I assume), I share with my patients that which I think I should, but not all that I might surmise, at least not at first. Patients and doctors hide and share in different ways, and for different reasons.

Sometimes sooner, sometimes later, with rage or with acceptance, politely or angrily, a patient with a chronic illness recognizes that her life is restricted, that there will be unpredictable flare-ups and remissions, and there likely will be withdrawal of families, spouses, and friends. Patients with chronic illnesses learn to protect themselves against the insensitivities of others, and against doctors who pretend to have answers that cannot possibly be known.

Sooner or later a doctor shares or hides information according to his guesses about what and when the patient needs or wants to know. The doctor balances realism and optimism when giving bad news and tries to sustain optimism when there is no hope at all. Neither the patient nor the doctor can be certain that the message intended is the one that will be heard.

Do people—doctors and patients, or anyone in a formal interaction in which one party is supplicant to the other—ever talk without using hidden messages? My wager is no. It is human nature for both parties to be optimistic in medical discussions, to hide deep fears, sidestep areas of conversation one or the other has signaled to be off limits, and not to hurt needlessly when there is no alternative to the pain.

If both parties try, they can, sometimes, hear the music in the words. Doctors may sense where a patient's weaknesses reside, they may intuit and uncover tricks that patients use to hide embarrassing information, they may probe gently into sensitive areas when there is clear need to elicit the answer. Patients can do the same with their doctors.

It is not so hard. Noting a glance in the wrong direction or a change of posture or tone, I can ask in a calm, even humorous, way, "Are you lying to me now?" Often the answer is a frank and unembarrassed, "Yes," followed by mention of what had been hidden. Unspoken fears do come to light.

Alida and I ended our book with this point: Every person has an inner strength. It is the doctor's duty to find its source. It is also a doctor's duty to let some questions stay unanswered and to anticipate that another answer, given by either doctor or patient, may be misunderstood. It is a doctor's duty to admit error if such has been made or to argue that, this time, I am right. It takes reading of eyes and of verbal tone. It takes an ability to hear the music of an out-of-context French phrase in the final stanza of a barely comprehensible, but famous, American poem.

26. To Teach the Lesson

It took me a long while to allow uncertainty a place in my world.

Then, pedagogue that I am, I decided to add the concept of uncertainty to my seminar course for the medical students.

This was not a good idea. The students were young, and at the beginning of their training. They knew only a little about only a few diseases. How could I tell them that they would never know enough? They needed to hear things that were more simple, not more complex. They wanted to hear about a world in which facts are certain, and they told me so.

I asked my colleagues if they knew a better time or way to teach about uncertainty. For the most part they agreed that the topic is important; they did not answer my question. At a curriculum committee meeting I talked about teaching uncertainty—same result. However, a colleague did say in that meeting that, in ten minutes, I had taught him everything important he had not heard in medical school but wished he had.

So I asked him, the committee, and later my colleagues, in hallways and staff meetings, if they knew of a better way and when to transmit this message to doctors-in-training. Each time the answer was a shrug and a blank stare. Yes, my colleagues said, the lesson is important. No, they said, we do not know how to teach it.

Perhaps the lesson is not for the young but for those further on. Perhaps it is a lesson for patients as well. Of course: It is a lesson for patients, too. But I still have no answer to my question, and there is no doubt that uncertainty must be taught.

In my world of chronic disease, as tests fail to define a problem, or as medicines work in unexpected and sometimes perverse ways, most patients eventually learn: Uncertainty remains part of my life. Thoughtful doctors, over time, begin to understand that, when diseases do not match their textbook descriptions, and when the illnesses of patients with purportedly the same diagnosis evolve in different ways, or when new and unexpected things appear, that we are at an unknown place on the trajectory of knowledge and an unknown distance on the arrow of Time. Recognizing the difference between what is surely known and that which is only surmised, we can talk about what we do not know with our patients. Doctors and patients alike can accept uncertainty, so long as surprises are few, we are open and honest, and we both continue to try. Can every doctor accept uncertainty? I cannot answer the question, except to say that the answer must be yes.

I know that some doctors cannot accept uncertainty. I do not fault them. Most acute medical events require immediate, confident decisions. You do not want the person putting a nail into your fractured leg or threading a catheter to your heart to have second thoughts about what to do. But you do hope that, before starting the procedure, the doctor had considered and weighed all the available options before moving ahead.

Perhaps we can say this: For acute illness there is mostly certainty; for chronic illness, often uncertainty. Indeed, to accept or reject uncertainty is what separates one vision of medicine from another. From the point of view of the patient, knowledge of uncertainty is what separates a "condition" from a "disease".

But this is simplistic. There is no precise boundary between acute and chronic. Remove the appendix, a scar remains, perhaps to cause future pain. Splint the fracture, the bone is never quite as good as it once was; perhaps a limp will remain. Survive the heart attack, take medications for the rest of your life. Acute sometimes become chronic. Chronic always begins as acute. In medicine, it is not a matter of uncertainty, *yes* or *no*.

It is instead a matter of uncertainty, little or much. Quantitative, not qualitative.

I had asked my colleagues, When is the best time to teach uncertainty? The question is still unanswered. Or perhaps this is part of the answer: Some doctors may never need to know. Some patients never want to know. If, patient or doctor, you know only acute illness, if you never have to face chronic illness, you can live in a world of certainty.

On the other hand, if, doctor or patient, your world is that of chronic illness, you have no choice. Uncertainty permeates your world. Doctors who care for patients with chronic illness must think, intuitively or explicitly, about uncertainty. They must give it a quantitative weight. Patients must live with uncertainty. Journalists, granting committees, and voluntary agencies should understand that simple, unnuanced descriptions do not apply to chronic illness. Criteria and guidelines committees should know that, even in the Internet age, diagnoses can be uncertain.

Omnipresent, not invalidating, uncertainty does not excuse inaction. It opens a doorway to an imaginative mind. It encourages innovation. When uncertainty is described and weighed, qualified and quantitated, doctors and patients can use it and manage it as they make their plans.

I had intended my course to teach about chronic illness and about the effect of Time. I discovered that, instead, I taught about uncertainty.

But perhaps the concepts, Time and Uncertainty, are really one, so in choosing to talk about Time I had chosen the correct theme after all. If you begin with the concept that today is a very brief moment of a very long Arrow of Time you will understand how evanescent is what we consider certain. Tomorrow's knowledge will supplement today's, and the elements of certainty will change. What we, doctor or patient, administrator or public, can do is act on what we do know now, articulate and quantify, name and weigh what we do not know, and use information about both the known and the unknown to make the best decisions that we can.

27. What is the Goal?

What is the patient's goal when she consults a doctor? Obviously, it is to feel well again. Does she achieve that goal by hearing a diagnosis or by prompting an open-minded inquiry into the mechanism (the process, how it came about) of the complaint? By hearing the problem's name, or by accepting treatment from someone who gave thoughtful consideration to how her suffering came to be? If the former, you think the way many scientists, administrators, and policy makers think about medicine—the name sufficiently explains all. If the latter, the name is just a descriptor, a handle that gives you first grasp to something much larger. If the latter, you think like a doctor.

For a doctor, precise diagnosis is not the most important goal, possibly not even an achievable aim. It is a word, a testable hypothesis, an embarkation point, a label used to validate an action to take. The hypothesis about the process is important. Its name is not.

Scientists consider diagnoses to be facts; they work backward: From this starting point (a mouse with a diagnosis), they ask, what mechanisms can we discern, or what treatments work? Practicing doctors think of diagnoses as working hypotheses, working in forward time, testing ideas and evaluating the results. A bedside diagnosis is a testable hypothesis about a single individual. A scientist makes hypotheses about groups that have pre-defined diagnoses. A physician commits an (often irreversible, potentially consequential) action to the hypothesis. A scientist commits less; if the hypothesis fails, he can vary the experiment and try again. To scientists who direct laboratory experiments or clinical trials a diagnosis is the single fact from which the investigation begins, so they discard outliers and exclude those who do not fit the pre-defined rules. A diagnosis at the bedside is a guess, subject to change; it applies to all, not just to those whose symptoms fit the rules.

.

28. What is the Lesson?

I began my journey with a question, How do I teach medical students about chronic illness?

This is my answer: The defining feature of chronic illness is uncertainty. I will teach the students to see it, define it, measure it, and place it in a context of time. I will teach them to turn uncertainty into a tool, to manage it, to live comfortably with it, and to include it as they make plans. I must teach this lesson also to patients, families, physicians, insurers, and administrators. And I must teach this as well: We need a common language to discuss this concept. We need to agree about the role of uncertainty, to negotiate a common ground.

Arrogance will stand in our way.

Advances in molecular biology sustain arrogance. Belief in the power of single molecules (molecular determinism) posits that the cause of most chronic illnesses is just one, or maybe just a few, abnormal molecules. The suspect molecules may come from the genome, the microbiome, the metabolome, or the epigenome—there are different views.[17] Wherever it lies, when the molecule is abnormal a critical biological process will fail, symptoms will follow, and the afflicted person will consult a doctor. The doctor will see a pattern of signs and symptoms, assign a diagnosis name, and prescribe a remedy targeted to the abnormal molecule. The remedy will bypass the process or repair the molecule. The symptoms will abate; health will return. This is the molecular determinists' theory.

Molecular determinists do not distinguish between diagnosis and abnormal process. Practicing doctors do.

Molecular determinists do permit incomplete forms of illnesses, overlapping illness, or diagnoses that change type over time. If you are a molecular determinist, the strange evolution of Milagros' and Anna's illnesses and the unconnected multiple ills that afflicted Amirah and Dale simply cannot be. The clinical observations must be wrong; the testing must be incorrect. If they were mice, or if they were considered for a clinical trial Milagros and Anna and Amirah would be excluded because they do not fit the pre-determined rule. Doctors conclude that

---

[17] The genome consists of any part of the body's DNA or RNA that controls a heritable factor. The microbiome is the body of bacteria that normally reside in or on the body, as in the intestinal tract or the skin. The metabolome is the set of biochemical processes that determine metabolism, particularly of body fat and sugar. The epigenome indicates the end products of processes that determine how strongly (or weakly) a gene exerts its effect.

what they observe is not error but an indicator that our science is still too primitive to understand. They see diagnoses as changing, mutable, processes that take place in instant clock, calendar, and generational time. Mysteries remain. We have far to go in our transit on the Arrow of Time.

Even without future knowledge can do better today. We can point out, quantitatively and qualitatively, the social, environmental, economic, personal, and emotional variables that contribute to a patient's problem. We can seek to know how the variables change over extended Time. We can focus more on process and less on cause. We can intercalate the unknown with the known as we think. Uncertainty is an invitation to learn.

Comfortable with uncertainty, we free ourselves of arrogance. Accepting that there are things we do not know, we free ourselves to imagine a larger world.

29. Note to Administrators: A Diagnosis is Not an Answer

Uncertainty about what?

Well, uncertainty about *diagnosis*.

Diagnosis, a venerated word, assumed to connote fact, but only a descriptive noun. A mere description, tentative, ephemeral, and mutable, a fulcrum, an hypothesis, not an answer.

I confess. I am making a political argument. I argue that today's focus on precision medicine is misguided.

Some will think me a troglodyte—how could I disparage the most advanced scientific knowledge ever to exist?

I understand that, for some small parts of medicine—some genetic diseases, a few infections, a few malignancies— precision medicine has had brilliant triumphs. But the triumphs are limited (not limitless). I believe that we will improve our concepts, our patient-physician dialogue, and our health care policies only by agreeing that today's knowledge is incomplete, only by acknowledging, understanding, and managing the uncertainty that remains.

This is my message: Sometime in the distant future "precision medicine" may apply to a majority of patients; it does not now. Uncertainty is ubiquitous, not only regarding biologic processes but also about those social, environmental, and other unmeasured externalities that determine how each individual patient fares. Your (you administrators) pretend-precise codes, guidelines, and algorithms prevent our including uncertainty in our plans. If you claim a level of precision that we cannot achieve you mislead the public: The first deception. It would be better to acknowledge how much we do not know, to accept the existence of uncertainty in your rules.

The clinical world contains un-mouse-like differences of sex, race, age, personal habits, finances, past experiences and beliefs, variables that influence the outcomes of illness as much as does its biology. A science laboratory can be precise; not so the messy human world. To ignore the effects of external human influences, to apply without qualification "facts" gleaned from mice to remedies for men—that is a second deception.

A third is to ignore that human diagnoses take place in extended time and that they change. I hope that the patients' tales in this book make this point clear.

Insurers, hospitals, policy makers, and patients themselves ask doctors to assign precise diagnoses, which the doctors do not themselves believe, a fourth deception.

The fifth and final deception is to believe that a specific diagnosis describes all persons afflicted with that illness. Doctors disagree; patients and doctors choose different health priorities; unmeasured aspects of personal interaction (the music of the words) influence decisions. Healthcare systems cannot assume that patient-doctor interactions are alike, or that an average for a population informs the care of an individual.

In my future utopia, we doctors will talk to our patients about the disease processes rather than about diagnoses. We will talk about context, Time, and variability. We will tell them what we do and do not know. We will individualize, not aggregate, patient care, and we will include socioeconomic, psychologic, environmental, and other contextual factors as well as the biologies of genes, cells, and microbes. Flexibility will supplant rigidity, and our imaginations will be more free.

30. What Proust Taught Me About Uncertainty

Each of us lives by quotations that we deem wise. For some of us, the quotations come from the movie *"The Godfather"*. For others they come from the Bible, the Founding Fathers, or the Constitution. My quotations come mostly from Proust's multivolume novel, *In Search of Lost Time*.

At the very end of the last volume Proust wrote, "If at least enough time is left to me to finish my work, I would describe there how men occupy a place... much larger than that (so restricted) that belongs to them in space... in Time."[xix]

In Search of Lost Time is (for him) about the process of preparing to write, or (for me) about how we learn to learn. On its face that premise seems exceedingly dull, but the journey that led to my writing this book is similar to that which Proust describes. Exploring one concept (how to manage chronic illness), I discovered a much larger one (how to manage uncertainty). I did not plan to emulate Proust—that would have been outrageously pretentious for me to do. But I do see parallels.

I had prepared a medical school course, the focus of which was Time. I taught that doctors think that they can predict, but in truth they only guess, what a patient's future will be. I taught that the rules that govern illness keep changing, and that certainty is constrained by our place both in space and in Time. I also taught that certainty is not a decision's most important quality.

As I taught, I began to see that we can include uncertainty in our decision-making. We can name and count the things that we comfortably know together with those that we know to be uncertain. We can listen for hidden messages. We can see the lines that connect cause to result. We can plan for events that occur simultaneously in instant, clock, calendar, and generational time. We can admit when we don't know.

I began to understand the process as I wrote about understanding the process.

The quotation from Proust that I cited above begins, "If at least enough time is left to me to finish my work…." The line sounds like he is accepting his mortality. He is not. He is accepting that he will not be able ever to complete some very big tasks. It means that uncertainty is inevitable.

Inevitable because we occupy a very small place on the infinitely long arrow of Time.

For my part, if enough time is left to me to finish my work, I will say that I can now live comfortably with uncertainty. If I am successful, I will teach that comfort to my students, to my patients, and to you.

Epilogue

Today we understand how illnesses work; we expect our doctors to make clear diagnoses. This is an age of precision medicine. Diagnostic uncertainty, the prestigious Institute of Medicine says, is error—correctable error—they say.[xx]

No (I say). Not correctable. No, not error.

Or maybe correctable—if what was error in 1917 (no antibiotics, just beginning to understand heart attacks) is no longer mystery in 2017 (but people still die of heart attacks, and many germs are now resistant to our antibiotics).

Diagnostic uncertainty is not error. Of course any doctor can be wrong, can misread the clues a patient offers, can misinterpret the results of tests, or can misuse a medication. I call those mishaps mistakes. Error is different. Error is to choose wrongly among *knowable* options. When the options include things that cannot be contemporaneously known—that (for the doctor in the early twentieth century) in half a century there will be an antibiotic that cures tuberculosis, that the lady of the camellias need not die—uncertainty is one of the acceptable options. It is a fully valid choice. To be self-importantly certain is error.

What is diagnostic uncertainty? The answer depends on how you define *diagnosis*. Diagnosis is "the process of determining by examination the nature and circumstances of a diseased condition,"[xxi] an Internet dictionary says.

The *process* of determining. Not the determination itself. Not the name. Not the cause. *How* an illness happened. Not *why* it happened. Not *what* it is.

You flip a switch, a light bulb shines. The snow that fell, the river that turns the waterwheel, generator that turns the water power to electricity, the wires, transformers, switches, and bulbs, all the small but critical pieces must work in concert to produce the light. Process does not tell us *why* the snow first fell or *what* the purpose of light may be. *Why* and *what* are absolutes, mysteries, subjects of religion, topics that *process* does not broach.

Between *why* and *what* is *how*, the prosaic part. *How* is the true subject of medicine, the small, sometimes nearly invisible points that doctors target to intervene. In medicine *process* has name. That name is *diagnosis*, a mere detail. Each and every process element that leads to that name is important, not the process' name.

* * * * *

This will sound curmudgeonly.

Once long ago I could justify my order for a medical test, or my reason for admitting a patient to a hospital, by writing this diagnosis in a patient's chart: "*r/o*" (shorthand for *rule out*) followed by my best guess.

R/o meant my diagnosis was tentative. If a patient complained of chest pain, I could write on my order or in the chart "*r/o MI*". By that little abbreviated note I told other doctors, administrators, and payers that, at that moment in the ER, I suspected myocardial infarction, MI, a medical name meaning heart attack.

Hours or days later, when the tests returned or something about the patient changed, I could update the admitting diagnosis. On day one the admitting diagnosis was *r/o MI*; on day three or five or it changed to *angina pectoris*, or *pleurisy*, or *rib fracture*, or *MI confirmed*. *R/o MI* had honestly and accurately justified the tests, the transfer to the ICU, and the medications I had prescribed. The chart was contemporary. You could watch my thoughts evolve in real time.

Today's computerized charts have no *r/o* diagnoses. There are no codes for uncertainty. If I see a patient with chest pain today I will choose among 31 separate codes for MI or other codes for rib fracture or pleurisy. For (the administrative, not the medical) purposes of charting and billing, the first code I click on will automatically populate all subsequent chart notes, prescriptions, and rendered bills, a computer-driven name, whether best guess or irrefutable fact, emblazoned at the top of each page, to mislead future readers until the end of time.

Curmudgeonly, I said. The old ways were better.

* * * * *

In the American presidential election of 2016 Donald Trump lost the popular vote but won enough Electoral College votes to become President. One doesn't really know what he will do, but he promised to repeal the Affordable Care Act ("ObamaCare") and to privatize Medicare. The possibilities are frightening. If these promises come to pass, my concerns about diagnostic certainty and uncertainty will still obtain. They will be meaningful for the long-term concept of medical science; they will still apply to the rest of the westernized world. But for the United States, diagnostic uncertainty will, for the short term, be a small concern. The big concern will be whether the disabled will have medical care at all.

My career started before Medicare and Medicaid came to be. I reminisced about these times in a book I once wrote. Here is what I wrote about the days when I was a medical intern:

> *I saw patients who waited until the last possible minute to come for help because they were ashamed that they could not pay the bills. I saw a husband of fifty years sell his car, his house, and everything else of value to provide custodial care for a wife disabled by stroke. I saw couples divorce so that the well, surviving spouse might keep a house and retain some control over a future life alone after the ill one was gone. What I did not see then, but did later, when I rode the police ambulance, and even later when I worked in small mining villages in West Virginia, were the people who chose, even those with treatable diseases, to die unattended because they could not afford care at all.*

Medicare and Medicaid became law in the 1960s. Then, in the 1980s, President Reagan, accusing "welfare queens," imposed sudden, severe restrictions on these programs. I wrote about these times, too:

> *The mechanism of termination* [from Medicaid coverage] *was cruel. It did not require those patients to prove why they should remain covered. Instead, they were first removed from the rolls and then asked to prove (in person) why they should be reinstated— not an easy job if you depend on a wheelchair for transportation,*

do not speak English, have a mental disability, or are discouraged
by long lines, churlish clerks, and constantly busy telephones.

To get Medicaid coverage again, even those who had been disabled
for years had to prove their eligibility anew. Many of my medically
stable patients delayed their clinic appointments or stopped coming
to see us altogether because they were physically and socially too
weak to speak in their own defense. Some returned by ambulance
when they ran out of medicine and became so ill that, in
desperation, their families or the police brought them back to us,
much sicker than they had ever been before. Despite the risk, that
ploy worked, because it was easy to reinstate a patient
hospitalized in an emergency to Medicaid.[xxii]

In 1965 Medicare and Medicaid had become law. Spouses no
longer had to divorce or declare bankruptcy. I moved to
another hospital when my training ended. Thanks to Medicaid,
my poor patients could (and did) go with me. Thanks to
Medicaid, they had the personal freedom regarding health care
that only the rich had enjoyed before.

Reagan's cutbacks in the 1980s were a painful but fortunately
transient, reminder of the bad days. The programs were by no
means perfect. Some people remained without medical
insurance. In 2010 ObamaCare began, and 23,000,000 more
Americans gained access to medical care.[xxiii]

If the new president's promises come true, the patients I describe in this book will be cast aside once again. Lacking personal wealth, those with chronic illnesses will have no defense. Disabled, they will lose their jobs, health insurance, and access to care. Once again they will be again hidden in back rooms, cared for by children or grandchildren or by no one at all, as they were before Medicare and Medicaid, as I saw as a Public Health Service officer in West Virginia in the 1960s, or abandoned in unheated tenement rooms, as I saw as a doctor in a police ambulance in New York. At best a few may cadge care, provided off the books by sympathetic doctors, as in Reagan's time.

Darwinian. The fit will survive. The disabled will not.

* * * * *

I see two problems.

The first is political, temporary, solvable: Will this nation agree to protect those who are chronically ill? I am optimistic that the answer is yes. Half a century ago we created Medicare and Medicaid. A quarter century ago – after a brief moment of disarray – these programs survived an attack not unlike that of today. With strong public support and societal compassion, I believe that common sense will prevail. Of course I worry about this, but the President's promise to repeal the Affordable Care Act is not my highest concern.

The second problem is the one that I fear. It is an intellectual problem, long term, also solvable. It is this challenge: To correct the mindset of doctors, patients, and public that gives priority to medical certainty and that insists that medical questions must have clearly wrong or clearly right answers. To correct the mindset that does not allow a defined place for uncertainty. A defined place that has a boundary, a weight, and a name. I hope we can correct this mindset for, if we are not free to ask questions, we cannot advance. But if we can name and quantify that which we do not understand, we will at least know how and what to ask.

Author's note

All patients described in these pages are real, but I have changed their names to protect their privacy. Similarly, although I have used quotation marks to describe certain conversations as they happened, the quotation marks represent a literary device rather than an indication of exactness, since I reconstructed the conversations from memory long after they took place. The spirit and gist of the quotations are, however, correct.

Acknowledgements

It is nearly impossible to thank all the people whose wisdom, advice, concerns, and random thoughts contributed to this book. Those named below represent a fraction of those on whom I relied.

First, of course, are all the patients who shared their thoughts and fears with me over several decades. Your allowing me to participate in the most intimate parts of your lives has both informed me and made me humble. Though for privacy reasons I cannot name you, you are my heroes.

Through conversations, example, wisdom, and friendship, my professional colleagues have contributed much to my way of thinking and often directly commented in many helpful ways. Among these are David Sachar, Doruk Erkan, Alana Levine, Steven Paget, and Peggy Crow. As I thought through some of these ideas in teaching medical students, Carol Storey-Johnson, from the Dean's Office, and Greg McDermott and Lester Zambrana, as students, offered important insights and, often, original new observations.

Alida Brill, with whom I had co-authored an earlier book, and Joe Spieler reviewed and commented on several earlier drafts of this book and helped shape it in its final form, as did my brother, Richard Lockshin and his wife, Zahra Zakeri. Jane, my life partner and wife, saw and critiqued every word many times over; her influence is unmeasurable; I have dedicated this book to her.

Conversations with Barbara Volcker led to the ideas about the meaning of diagnosis and the role of long-term thinking in patient-doctor relationships that form the heart of this book. The generous support of her widower, Paul Volcker, has allowed her wishes to develop and to be applied to a larger world.

Much of what I wish to convey was birthed in conversations with, and presentations before patient groups convened by, our hospital's remarkable social services department, headed by Roberta Horton, ably assisted by Su Jin (Suzy) Kim and My-Lan Tran. Others, in other hospital divisions, who also helped me form ideas are Nadine Spring and (now young physician) Kamini Doobay.

For all the others whom I neglected to mention, my apologies. I am grateful to you nonetheless.

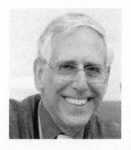

About the Author

Dr. Michael D. Lockshin is one of America's preeminent experts in the long-term care of chronically ill patients. He is a pioneer in solving health-care issues that arise with the illnesses on which he has done his most renowned research – systemic lupus erythematosus, antiphospholipid antibody syndrome, and other autoimmune diseases which especially afflict women. He is regularly listed in New York Magazine's Best Doctors series and in Castle Connolly's America's Top Doctors Books. In November 2008, the New York Arthritis Foundation honored Dr. Lockshin with its Lifetime Achievement Award.

Currently, Dr. Lockshin is Director of the **Barbara Volcker Center for Women and Rheumatic Disease at the Hospital for Special Surgery** and Professor of Medicine and Obstetrics-Gynecology at Weill Cornell Medicine in New York.

Dr. Lockshin is a past editor-in-chief of Arthritis & Rheumatism, the official publication of the American College of Rheumatology and the leading journal in the field worldwide.

A world renowned researcher, Dr. Lockshin has authored over 300 research papers, book chapters, and books and has edited several conference proceedings and books. His book for the general reader, Guarded Prognosis: A Doctor and His Patients Talk about Chronic Disease and How to Cope With It, was published by Hill and Wang, a division of Farrar, Straus and Giroux, in 1998. His last book for general audience, Dancing At The River's Edge: A Patient and Her Doctor Negotiate a Life With Chronic Illness (Schaffner Press, Inc.)

was published in 2009. It is a personal dual memoir, written in collaboration with long-time patient Alida Brill.

Dr. Lockshin has held senior management positions at The National Institutes of Health in Bethesda, Maryland. He served first as Director of the Extramural Program of the National Institute of Arthritis and Musculoskeletal and Skin Diseases and then as Acting Director of the Institute. This Institute is responsible for U.S. government research funding in the fields of rheumatology and dermatology. He also served as Senior Advisor to the Director at the NIH's Warren G. Magnuson Clinical Center.

Prior to joining NIH, Dr. Lockshin was a Professor of Medicine at Weill Cornell Medical College and attending rheumatologist at the Hospital for Special Surgery and New York Hospital. Dr. Lockshin interned and did his residency at Bellevue Hospital and Memorial Hospital for Cancer and Allied Diseases; his fellowship in Rheumatic Diseases at Columbia Presbyterian Medical Center in New York City.

Dr. Lockshin is a recognized leader in the field of rheumatology. He chaired the American Board of Internal Medicine Committee on Rheumatology, the committee which writes the exam that certifies all US rheumatologists in the subspecialty. He has held national offices and chaired committee at the Arthritis Foundation and the American College of Rheumatology (ACR.) He chaired the ACR Visual Aids Committee that produced the first Clinical Slide Collection. This collection is used by rheumatologists around the world to illustrate rheumatic diseases and their clinical and biological manifestations. He was the first chairman of the ACR standing Committee on Rheumatological Practice which investigated quackery in the field. He has served on the editorial boards of Arthritis & Rheumatism, Journal of Rheumatology, Lupus, American Journal of Reproductive Immunology, and other journals.

Dr. Lockshin is an original thinker who has brought together researchers from disparate fields to solve problems in the rheumatic disease area. He convened the first international Conference on Pregnancy and Rheumatic Disease and the first ever Conference on Gender, Biology, and Human Disease.

He was a member of the Institute of Medicine Committee on Understanding the Biology of Sex and Gender Differences, its Committee to Review the CDC Anthrax Vaccine Safety and Efficacy Research Program, its Health Sciences Policy Board, and its Committee on (NIH) Centers of Excellence Programs.

Dr. Lockshin graduated cum laude from Harvard College with a BA in history and literature. He received his MD from Harvard Medical School.

For more information see: www.MichaelLockshin.com.

Praise for Dr. Lockshin's books

Guarded Prognosis: A Doctor and His Patients Talk about Chronic Disease and How to Cope with It

Kirkus Reviews
Guarded Prognosis: A Doctor and His Patients Talk about Chronic Disease and How to Cope with It

Using his patients' personal stories to illustrate dramatically how medical care once worked and how it works today, a concerned and caring physician makes clear just why he fears the current system has a very poor prognosis. Director of the Center for Women and Rheumatic Disease at the Hospital for Special Surgery in New York, Lockshin specializes in lupus, a chronic disease that affects every organ in the body and brings its patients into contact with all segments of the medical-care system. Drawing on some 35 years of medical experience, he writes knowingly and sympathetically of patients who need long-term, expensive care, whose problems may require speedy treatment by specialists. In doing so, he questions how well such individuals would fare in a system where primary-care doctors act not as their patients' advocates but as gatekeepers, deciding who will have access to what kind of care. He acknowledges that cost is at the heart of the medical-care crisis, but points out that this cost comes largely from common, chronic, and crippling diseases. Lockshin outlines what he perceives as the elements of an ideal system and calls for a vigorous public debate over the issues, which, he notes, seem medical but are social and political as well. He argues that decision-making criteria concerning health-care resources and spending must include compassion as well as cost-benefit. The questions he raises about cost cutting, rationing of care, doctor-patient privacy, and individual needs and rights are ones that deserve careful consideration. An able spokesman for the poor and chronically ill, those whose voices he believes are seldom heard in the debate over health policy in this country, he has given us stories to remind us that abstract policies affect individuals who could be us or those we love. — Copyright ©1998, Kirkus Associates, LP. All rights reserved.

Publishers Weekly
Guarded Prognosis: A Doctor and His Patients Talk about Chronic Disease and How to Cope with It

With 35 years' experience as a physician, Lockshin remembers the days before Medicare, Medicaid and HMOs. Working particularly with lupus patients, he has accrued vast knowledge of chronic illness, insurance and hospital administration. Here, in the voice of a caring doctor whose primary concern is always the welfare of his patients, Lockshin provides moving human case histories that illustrate current issues and dilemmas in American medicine. His prognosis is bleak, as he details how the personal welfare of individuals and their families is often ignored by a system obsessed with numbers and, ultimately, "comfortable profits." Lockshin finds that, in particular, the elderly, the poor and those with chronic illnesses are not well served by the number-crunching approach of insurance companies and hospital administrations. He observes that limiting the number and kinds of tests and procedures, the length of hospital stays and access to specialists keeps costs down in the short term, but drastically reduces the quality of care and often ends up costing more later. In this enlightening and frightening book, Lockshin carefully considers all sides to his arguments and, finally, offers hope that beneficial compromise is still possible. Copyright 1998 Reed Business Information, Inc.

Booklist

Guarded Prognosis: A Doctor and His Patients Talk about Chronic Disease and How to Cope with It

The subtitle tells much more about this book than the title. For doctors do not treat aggregates of patients, they treat individual humans. Lockshin argues that governments, insurance companies, hospitals, and HMOs should listen to individuals rather than the impersonal figures aggregates produce. Many of Lockshin's patients have lupus, arthritis, or scleroderma. Since those diseases affect different patients in different ways, Lockshin's emphasis on the individual makes sense; each person's sense of health priorities, he says, should be carefully considered when choosing a treatment program. Lockshin draws a clearcut distinction between medicine and science: the former deals primarily with individuals, the latter with theories and groups. Since HMOs have come into the picture, many doctors are being forced to think of each potential patient in terms of whether this treating of this person is going to be an occasion of profit or of loss, and he asks, "Are you sure that you know for whom your doctor works?" William Beatty.

Chapters.indigo.ca

Guarded Prognosis: A Doctor and His Patients Talk about Chronic Disease and How to Cope with It

From Our Editors Like James Herriott, Oliver Sacks and Lewis Thomas, Michael Lockshin teaches us about illness and health by telling stories about medicine. His stories focus not on disease, but the risks of the health care system. He demonstrates the heartbreaking, horrifying and hilarious situations patients and doctors must deal with – the kind not found in insurance company formulas. Not only does Guarded Prognosis honour the ill and those who care for them, it shows exactly how health care could be more efficient, less costly and more humane. From http://www.chapters.indigo.ca/

Booknews

Descrying the survival of the fittest mentality of Health Maintenance Organizations (HMOs), this New York specialist in rheumatic diseases (e.g. rheumatoid arthritis and lupus) and onetime director of National Institute of Health programs makes a cogent plea using case histories and analysis for ensuring a health care safety net and healthy doctor-patient partnership for all<--> including the elderly and those with costly chronic conditions. Annotation c. by Book News, Inc., Portland, Or.

"Brill's writings and Lockshin's writings . . . are poetic, revealing, insightful, and at times shocking in their honest and frank discussion of aspects of chronic disease that are rarely brought out into the open." —*New England Journal of Medicine*

"*Dancing at the River's Edge* . . . is about the trials and tribulations of chronic disease . . . you ought to get a copy and read it. You won't be able to put it down once you pick it up." —Paul A. Volcker, former Federal Reserve chairman

"A deeply personal exploration on both sides of the medical scene—the patient who suffers and strives to retain her 'self,' and the physician who struggles to maintain a balance between knowing the truth while attempting to understand its implications." —Virginia Ladd, president and executive director, American Autoimmune Diseases Related Association

"An extraordinary meditation on illness—a poetic, powerful and groundbreaking work that illuminates the resilience and strength of the human spirit." —David Isay, executive director, Storycorps, and editor, *Listening Is an Act of Love*

"A must-read for anyone who has traveled to the 'other planet' that is chronic illness, or loves someone who is making this arduous journey . . . a life-affirming and deeply moving book." —Nancy Matsumoto, staff contributor, *People*; former contributor, *Health, Los Angeles Times, New York Times, Newsweek*, and *Time*; coauthor, *The Parents' Guide to Eating Disorders*

"A book unlike any other; this slim volume probes the intricacies of a magical relationship, that of a patient with her doctor. A heart-wrenching dialogue that carries profound and life-altering insights for us all." —Dr. David Sachar, Emeritus Clinical Professor of Medicine and Director Emeritus of the GI Division, Mount Sinai Medical School and Mount Sinai Hospital

"Whether you are doctor or patient, you see a bit of yourself in [this book]. . . . It demonstrates how profound the bond between doctor and patient can be—how much power it imparts." —Susan Golick, founder, S.L.E. Lupus Foundation

"Delves into the intricacies and intimacy of chronic illness . . . it illuminates the spirit. Important for those suffering from chronic illness and [their] families." —Lauren Shuler Donner, film producer, *You've Got Mail* and the X-Men series, a lupus patient

Dancing at the River's Edge is a beautiful book, both informative and moving, written from the heart by people who, through their interactions over the years, and through the conversation recorded in this book, know each other and themselves intimately. It is introspective, often poetic, always honest—the creation of "a meeting of minds and hearts...a peculiar kind of magic." Kathy Waller for Story Circle Book Reviews www.storycirclebookreviews.org/reviews/riversedge.shtml

This is an extraordinary and unique book - - a classic. It should be mandatory reading for all people with chronic medical and autoimmune conditions, the people who love them, as well as all medical students, residents, fellows and physicians. This amazing book does nothing less than define what it means to live with a chronic autoimmune disorder - - as seen through the eyes of the top rheumatologist in the world and a patient with a writing gift that allows her feelings and experiences to explode from the page. Stephen A. Paget, M.D. Physician-in-Chief Emeritus, Division of Rheumatology at Hospital For Special Surgery and the Joseph P. Routh Professor of Medicine and

Rheumatic Disease at the Weill Medical College of Cornell University and the New York Presbyterian Hospital.

ENDNOTES

[i] Butler, D. When Google got flu wrong. Nature 2013 (14 February) 494: 155-156.

[ii] Cited by Valle, D., Genetics, individuality, and medicine in the 21st century. Am J Hum Genet. Mar 2004; 74(3): 374–381, PMCID: PMC 1182248. Published online Feb 19, 2004.

[iii] Kavanagh, Julie. The Girl Who Loved Camellias: The Life and Legend of Marie Duplessis, New York:Knopf, 2013, location 3222/5226

[iv] T. S. Eliot, *Collected Poems 1909-1962*, Harcourt:Orlando, 1963, "The Love Song of J. Alfred Prufrock," p. 5.

[v] Frost, Robert. The Road Not Taken. http://www.bartleby.com/119/1.html, March 30, 2014

[vi] http://www.cdc.gov/nchs/icd/icd10cm_pcs_background.htm accessed July 19, 2014. ICD-9 lists 14,025 diagnoses and 3,824 procedures; ICD-10 69,828 diagnoses and 71,924 procedures.

[vii] December 29, 2013

[viii] http://www.healthcaredive.com/news/the-16-most-absurd-icd-10-codes/285737/#.U8kE6Y4SFek.mailto accessed July 19, 2014.

[ix] *Diseases:* Antiphospholipid syndrome; ankylosing spondylitis (separated from rheumatoid arthritis); neuromyelitis optica; Lassa fever; Ebola virus; HIV; Lyme disease; Norwalk virus; JC virus and progressive multifocal

leukoencephalopathy; Kaposi's sarcoma and HTLV-3; Jamaican paraparesis and HTLV-1; hepatitis C; EBV and Burkitt's lymphoma; molecular susceptibilities of certain cancers, like HER-2 in breast cancer and B-cell lymphomas; Spanish toxic oil syndrome; L-tryptophan toxicity; polonium poisoning; drug-induced lupus; amiodarone lung toxicity; non-ST-elevation myocardial infarction. *Technologies:* CT scans; MRI; MRA; PET scans; minimally invasive surgery, including arthroscopy, laparoscopy,and coronary bypass; total joint replacement; heart transplant; face transplant; hand transplant.

[x] Molecular biologists and other scientists often display complexity graphically. A common model consists of colored circles connected by lines, with groups of several circles together clustered within a dotted line. Imagine one of these clusters of circles. The circles vary in both size and color. The different sizes and the colors indicate strengths—quantities— of whatever one wants to show. Each circle represents some element, like the amount of a substance in blood, and those in clusters are related in some way. If one circle is very large it means that that substance has a large effect. If the circle is small, not so much. The colors represent a different kind of strength, like power to influence. For instance one color, say red, shows a strong positive influence, so a large red circle means there is a lot of something, and it has a strong influence. If the circle is light pink, it is present in the same amount, but its influence is less; if it is deep red, its influence is even more. If the circle is smaller but deep red, a smaller amount will still have an important effect: One can give numbers to the colors and the sizes and multiply the color by the size to understand the total effect. One can change to a different0 color, say blue,

to show an opposite effect. The deeper blue, the more whatever you are measuring is repressed.

Now connect some of these circles with lines. The lines will vary in width, thick lines meaning a tight connection between two circles, thin a loose connection. You can give numbers to the lines so that you can count and calculate the net effect of the color, the circle size, and the line thickness.

For the molecular biologists, a little circle may reflect the influence of a single gene, call one gene A and another gene B. By using the numbers assigned to the circles, their colors, and their connecting lines, one can calculate how much a change in, say, the function of gene A, will cause in the function of gene B.

[xi] Each scores three on the severity scale for symptoms/signs (weight 10) and each scores two on the severity scale for laboratory abnormalities (also weight 10), so each gets a total of 30 points for symptoms/signs plus 20 for laboratory, giving a total of 50. Had I used SLEDAI, they would also be equal, since SLEDAI counts these same elements. At this point SLEDAI and MDLLE would both predict similar prognoses.

[xii] In the Tuskegee experiments African American men were, without their knowledge, not treated for decades, to learn the "natural history" of untreated syphilis.

[xiii] Henrietta Lacks was the African American woman whose cancer cells were repeatedly taken without her knowledge and sold at high profit (to others) for tissue culture experiments. See Skloot, Rebecca, *The Immortal Life of Henrietta Lacks*, Crown Books, SBN 978-1-4000-5217-2.

xiv T.S. Eliot, *ibid*, p. 51

xv T.S. Eliot, *ibid*, p. 53

xvi http://www.poesie.net/nerval3.htm, accessed March 9, 2014

xviihttp://www.penguinclassics.ca/nf/shared/WebDisplay/0,,49012_1_10,0
0.html, searched December 29, 2013

xviii Brill A, Lockshin M. *Dancing at the River's Edge: A Patient and her Doctor
Negotiate Live with Chronic Illness.* Schaffner Press: Tucson, 2009

xix Proust M. *Le Temps retrouvé*, Paris:Gallimard, 1989, p. 353. Author's
translation.

xx National Academy of Sciences Institute of Medicine, Improving
Diagnosis in Health Care, Balogh EP, Miller BT, Ball JR, editors. The
National Academies Press: Washington, 2015, 369 pp. P. S-2.

xxi http://dictionary.reference.com/browse/diagnosis

xxii Lockshin, Michael D. *Guarded Prognosis*, 1998. New York:Hill & Wang, p
8 and p 174

xxiii
https://en.wikipedia.org/wiki/Patient_Protection_and_Affordable_C
are_Act searched November 26, 2016